Praise for UNBUTTONED

7/2009

"*Unbuttoned* is what every mom wishes she knew before she started on
the breastfeeding journey."

—Laura Berman Fortgang, author of *Living
Your Best Life* and *Now What?*

"This collection of essays struck home like a missile. Who knew that
so many other moms had walked my path of pride, frustration, pain,
and joy while breastfeeding? It's about time we shared our journeys
through humor and hope!"

—Deborah Roberts, network television journalist

"Lots of books tell you why you should breastfeed. Lots of books tell
you how to breastfeed. Not many books talk about why you *want* to
breastfeed. This one does, and in its 'show, don't tell' essays, it also delivers the real-life how-to."

—Trisha Thompson, executive editor,
Wondertime magazine

"Every woman who becomes a mother will recognize herself somewhere in *Unbuttoned*, which offers a wide range of intensely personal and sometimes political perspectives on breastfeeding. These personal essays—frank, funny, and profound—provide a welcome antidote to the bewildering array of how-to manuals and advice books that populate new mothers' shelves."

—Christina Baker Kline, author of *The Way*
Life Should Be and co-editor of *About Face*

"*Unbuttoned* is wonderful! As I read the essays, I experienced anew those special seasons of my life when I breastfed my own three sons, now grown. As one of the book's contributors so aptly describes it, nursing is 'God's reward, perhaps, for the hard work of motherhood.' "

—Kathy Peel, founder and CEO, Family Manager Coaching and
author of *The Busy Mom's Guide to a Happy, Organized Home*

UNBUTTONED

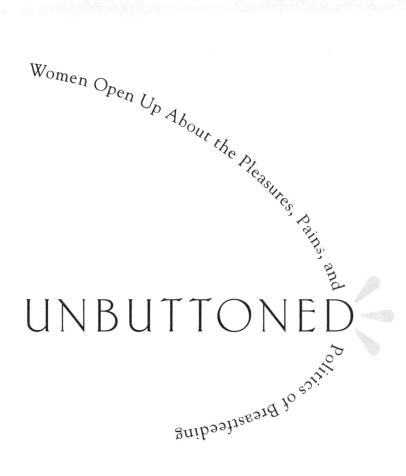

Women Open Up About the Pleasures, Pains, and Politics of Breastfeeding

UNBUTTONED

Edited by

Dana Sullivan and Maureen Connolly

THE HARVARD COMMON PRESS
Boston, Massachusetts

The Harvard Common Press
535 Albany Street
Boston, Massachusetts 02118
www.harvardcommonpress.com

Printed in the United States of America
Printed on acid-free paper

Library of Congress Cataloging-in-Publication Data
Unbuttoned : women open up about the pleasures, pains, and politics
of breastfeeding / edited by Dana Sullivan and Maureen Connolly.
    p. cm.
  ISBN 978-1-55832-397-1 (pbk.)
  1. Breastfeeding--Miscellanea. 2. Breastfeeding--Anecdotes.
3. Lactation--Miscellanea. 4. Lactation--Anecdotes. I. Sullivan,
Dana. II. Connolly, Maureen.
  RJ216.U33 2009
  649'.33--dc22
                                              2008034204

Special bulk-order discounts are available on this and other
Harvard Common Press books. Companies and organizations may
purchase books for premiums or resale, or may arrange a custom edition,
by contacting the Marketing Director at the address above.

Cover design by Night & Day Design
Cover photograph © Corbis
Text design by Jennifer Daddio

10 9 8 7 6 5 4 3 2 1

To Liam, Julia, and Carina:

You nourish me every day;
I am the luckiest mother in the world.
—DS

To Jack, Sean, and Henry:

May I always be able to feed
your hearts and souls.
—MC

CONTENTS

FOREWORD

Until we're pregnant, we have all sorts of feelings about our breasts: They're too big, too small, too saggy, too full, uneven, our favorite feature or the one we most wish to change. But during pregnancy, or shortly thereafter, the focus suddenly shifts from form to function. For some of us, this is the first time we've really considered what our breasts are designed to do: produce milk for babies.

The increase in breast size during pregnancy and after birth makes many women feel sexy, and knowing that their breasts are sustaining a life boosts many moms' self-esteem and sense of purpose. But there are also women who feel anything but sexy when nursing and lament the loss of their breasts as theirs alone. "I feel like a milk machine"—or worse, "a cow"—is how some women sum it up. Some moms are also disappointed by how their breasts perform—they seem unable to do the job they were made to do. That was me.

As the editor of BabyCenter, the Web's most popular destination for pregnancy and parenting information, I'd worked on hundreds of articles about the health benefits of nursing for babies and moms. To think about anything other than breast-feeding was blasphemy. Fast forward nine months, and I was in the throes of a serious breastfeeding drama. I had cracked and bleeding nipples, searing pain with latch-on, two cases of mas-titis, and thrush—all within the first six weeks. But I didn't throw in the towel. I felt I couldn't, and with each challenge I faced, my urge to go on strengthened. "You can't quit now," I told myself. "Look what you've been through already." I nursed my daughter until she was six months old—longer than I thought I could during the early days, but not long enough to satisfy the American Academy of Pediatrics or assuage my mommy guilt.

A lot of women have had similar experiences. One survey of BabyCenter moms showed that two out of three felt guilty about not breastfeeding or stopping too soon. As "beautiful and natural" as breastfeeding is, I've learned, it doesn't come easy for the vast majority of new moms.

Breastfeeding is consistently one of the top twenty search terms on BabyCenter, and it's one of the top five conversation topics in our online community. Clearly breastfeeding is some-thing that women feel compelled to talk about. In our recent poll on the subject, 21 percent of the women who responded told us that they were "surprised" by how much they enjoyed nursing. The flip side of that: 25 percent were surprised by how hard it is.

This book is about women facing their breastfeeding chal-lenges head on and making choices that only they can make. Each beautifully written, searingly honest story reminds me that no matter what your breastfeeding experience—or for-mula-feeding experience—you're not alone. So settle down—

with a babe in your arms or not—and let yourself be moved by this incredible collective of mothers who open their hearts and shirts to bare their poignant breastfeeding stories.

—Linda Murray
Editor-in-chief, BabyCenter.com

When *Unbuttoned* was conceived, one of us (Dana) was eighteen months into breastfeeding her third child, and the other (Maureen) was a few weeks into her third pregnancy. We initially wanted to write a "how-to" book about breastfeeding, given the breadth of experiences—both good and, well, challenging—that we'd had. But we discovered that even though there wasn't one book on the market that included everything we wanted to hear, there were several that pretty much covered the bases. And since breastfeeding is one of those topics that elicits a reaction, an opinion, or a story from almost every woman who has had a child—whether she has nursed or not—we realized that an anthology could allow room for many different points of view.

Ultimately, the amazing writers we found gave us more than we could have dreamed of, and they shared their intimate stories with humor, candor, pain, and elation. One writes about her experiences dating while lactating. Another *still* feels the need to defend her decision not to breastfeed, even though her oldest child is now a teenager. Weaning is treated comically in two essays, and in another with an aching that brought tears to our eyes. Readers will undoubtedly see the truth in both perspectives. Every writer's experience is unique, but the themes of wonder, frustration, and gratitude are universal.

Suzanne Schlosberg was convinced that we'd find a publisher for this book; thank you, Suzanne, for helping us find Bruce Shaw, president and publisher at The Harvard Common Press. Bruce "got" the idea behind this book right away—and took a chance by agreeing to publish the company's first anthology. Jane Dornbusch and the crew at The Harvard Common Press came up with the perfect title; our editor, Linda Ziedrich, was so very patient while the essays trickled in and made astute observations that polished each one of them. We are grateful to our agent, Kathleen Spinelli, who believed in the book from the beginning and kept us on track. Thank you to the editors and writers who so eagerly read advance galleys of the book and offered their thumbs-ups and public endorsements. Christina Baker Kline, we are also grateful for your insights on all things book publicity–related. Most of all, we wholeheartedly thank all the wonderful writers who agreed to collaborate with us on this project.

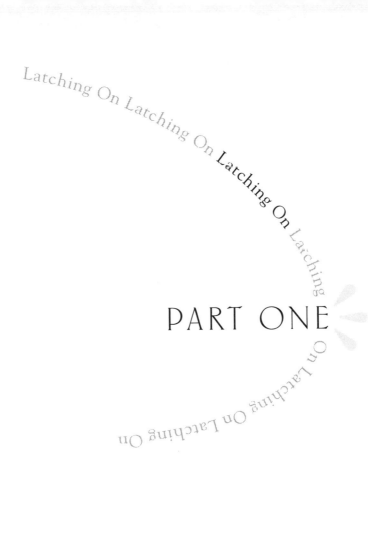

Latching On Latching On Latching On Latching On Latching On Latching On Latching On

PART ONE

THE WHOLE TRUTH (AND NOTHING BUT THE TRUTH)

Julia Glass

When my second son was about a week old, I phoned the pediatrician in tears. My darling baby was mauling me. He was getting the milk he needed—he was, as the experts put it, "thriving"—but he was clamping onto my breast like a toothless piranha on steroids.

Back then, Oliver's pediatrician was an impishly dashing Frenchman whose bedside manner was a captivating blend of charisma and candor, both extreme. So when I got him on the phone that day and said I was having a harder time with breastfeeding the second time around, he barked, "You do remembair zat EET URTS, do you not?"

I laughed. "Oh yes. That part I do remember."

"Good!" he exclaimed robustly. "Because eet does. Eet urts!" And then he told me how to give Oliver a crash course on infant table manners. I would get some relief—but lose zee pain? Not so fast, *chérie*.

My boys are now eleven and six, their nurturing at my breast a thing of the distant past, so I'd like to believe that the way women learn about breastfeeding is different now from the way it was in the final years of the last millennium. But something tells me that political correctness, New Age feminism, and the lacunae between medical specialties still conspire to perpetuate the fantasy of breastfeeding as something so patently instinctive, so obviously healthy, such an ideal melding of the earthy and the soulful, that it will come to the novice mother as easily as breathing oxygen comes to her baby. Which means that when breastfeeding goes from fantasy to reality, this is what it feels like: the rude surprise of a lifetime.

What's so ironic is that modern American women are, if anything, overprepared for childbirth and baby care. Every microminute of the normal (and abnormal) pregnancy is documented in book after book. Before the hallowed baby makes an entrance, we are encouraged to make "birth plans," to practice diapering and burping on dolls, to order straps and plugs and gates to childproof our homes, to learn infant CPR, to sign up in advance for Mommy-and-me music and fitness groups. We and our fetuses are probed, prodded, sonographed, injected, phlebotomized, Lamazed, and genetically parsed. With joy and trepidation, we buy the car seat, the crib, the bibs, the burp cloths, the wipes, the mobiles, the diaper rash ointment, the dozens of teeny-tiny T-shirts—oh, the things we buy!

All the while, our breasts discreetly fill and swell; our nipples pout and darken; the veins across our chests stand out like meandering rivers on a fragile antique map. We (and our mates) admire these changes and make raunchy jokes about sharing. But when—amid all that shopping—we stop to fantasize about the new intimacy our breasts will give us with our first babies, I'll bet most of us still foresee an instant state of grace. Who doesn't catch a grandiose glimmer of the halos surrounding the heads of all those serene Madonnas on Christmas cards, in Sunday school primers, sanctified in museums and churches alike?

The first time I was pregnant, I was the only woman I knew who worried about the nitty-gritty of nursing—but I had good reason. A few years before, I'd been treated for early-stage breast cancer. Because the cancer was hormone-receptor-negative, and because it had not recurred, the doctors gave my pregnancy their cautious blessing. For the sake of vigilance, my breast surgeon examined my breasts every two months until the birth.

As pregnancy progressed, my left breast began to change—but not the right, the "treated" breast, the one that had been sliced, diced, and nuked. A lumpectomy had left it only negligibly smaller than its cohort, so my doctors told me, early on, that it would probably come through in the end. By month seven, however, I had one breast resembling a shiny, eager torpedo and another that looked more like an old sock lost behind the hamper.

Would I be able to nurse with one functioning breast? Absolutely, said my doctors. ("Just think of twins," said my obstetrician gaily. "One spigot per kid!") But this did not assuage my anxiety—or my journalistic curiosity. What would it feel like to nurse? How would I *learn*? Both my obstetrician and my surgeon were men, but they were also fathers. "Don't worry about that now," they scoffed. "You'll do just fine." What they did not say was that, as far as they were concerned, my breasts had now entered the domain of the pediatrician . . . whom I had yet to meet.

Not satisfied, I began to grill my girlfriends. Nearly forty, I was arriving at motherhood late; most of my female peers had one or two children already. I knew by heart every one of their colorful, distinctly intrepid birth stories—all of which were re-cited anew, now that I would be joining the club. Strangely, though, I realized I hadn't heard much commentary on nursing. So I began asking.

Was I ever shocked when the first friend I asked burst out with something like this: "Oh God. I hated every minute. And when I called this breastfeeding hot line, they told me I needed to concentrate on 'bonding' with my daughter. If I did that, I'd automatically love it. Like I wasn't paying enough attention to her! I decided three months would be enough. I counted the days." Her husband, she disclosed, had been repelled by her difficulties with nursing; during one heated debate (fueled by sleeplessness, no doubt), he'd even accused her of having am-bivalent feelings toward nurturing their daughter. At the time, she had kept her shame, and the marital discord, entirely to herself.

Another woman I knew, a tough, droll Texan, took a philo-sophical tone when she confessed, "Well, I'd have to say that it hurt like hell. At first. And then it got better."

A mother I regard as Supermom of the Millennium said, "I made it three weeks, until I ended up in the emergency room, delirious with a high fever, my breasts engorged to the point where my son couldn't nurse at all. I had mastitis. They strapped me into a corset, gave me heavy-duty antibiotics, and told me my nursing career was over. I was relieved."

"I loved it," said another, "once I got past the cracking and bleeding."

The what?

Why, I asked my friends, hadn't they told me any of this before? Because each of them had assumed she was an excep-tion. Or a freak. Or a sissy. After all, the "experts" were happy to share with us in Faulkner-esque detail the nuclear wattage of a labor contraction—videos were shown, war stories told—so if breastfeeding was a challenge, wouldn't they be just as frank? Discussions of nursing might invoke, at worst, that all-purpose medical euphemism *discomfort*. In some warped scenarios, nursing was portrayed as a sort of "reward" after the ordeal of birth. (Here's another factoid the experts didn't tell us. It hurts more with each subsequent baby—not the nursing itself but the cramping triggered by the nursing, as your increasingly capacious uterus works harder to shrink back down. Just after Oliver was born, while I was still in the hospital, I mentioned this new sensation to a passing nurse. She explained what was happening, then said, "Oh, honey, you think it feels bad now? Wait till number *five*.")

From what I was hearing, the exception was not the woman tempted to quit this endeavor but the one who thought it was no big deal.

* *

Now, can I stop here to say that when I look back on breast-feeding my children, I am pierced with a tearful, intense nostalgia for the closeness, the joy, the animal love, all those glowy clichés—yes, even the Madonna-like grace—that I felt once we'd found our groove? It nearly broke my heart to wean them at six months—which I was compelled to do because of my medical history (clear mammograms cannot be taken of lactating breasts).

Does that seem absurd? The point is this: So many women I know quit nursing early, or suffered tense rifts with perplexed spouses, because no one had told them what to expect. From everything they had heard, they assumed that the pain would end at childbirth and the joy would begin at the breast. This was the promise behind the propaganda.

But there's a logical history to the propaganda. To begin with, pity the poor pediatric academies back in the eighties and nineties. They were in the business of eating their words. Big-time. Responsible American mothers who'd given birth during the postwar era of chemicals for better living—that is, the mothers of the mothers in my age group—fed their babies formula. Formula was milk engineered to uniform perfection: That's what their doctors told them. As my own mother, who grew up on a dairy farm, told me, "We were not mere cows, to be milked, for heaven's sake. We had evolved beyond that!" Those mothers went on to feed us, again with pride and medical approval, food prepared from kits and powders: Hamburger Helper, Jell-O 1-2-3, TV dinners, mashed potatoes in a box, everything canned, freeze-dried, reconstituted, powdered. Remember the macho panache of Tang?

Honestly, now, could you picture Jane Jetson holding Elroy or Judy to her naked breast? June nursing the Beav?

And then the seventies came rolling through town. Women rediscovered food as connected to nature, and for the first time they took a good look at their bodies (possibly because the clothes we wore over them in that era were so outrageously ugly). When I was in college, every young woman in the know was sure to own two books irrelevant to schoolwork: *The Moosewood Cookbook* and *Our Bodies, Ourselves.* Bring back butter and you'll never touch margarine again. Take off your bra and the breast will have its unmuzzled say. "What was I meant for?" it proclaimed.

Did those guys in the white coats have some explaining to

do! But changing approaches to public health is about as easy as parking an RV in midtown Manhattan. Yes, the academic baby doctors, the newest baby books, and La Leche League (referred to by every mother I knew as the Nursing Gestapo) were ardently chanting, "Breast is best!" But when confronted with a new mother sobbing at the pain of nursing, even the most urbane pediatricians would quietly advise her that formula was perfectly fine. After all, that's what *we* got, right? And what's the matter with us?

My first son and I were fortunate. At Alec's very first office checkup, the nurse practitioner who worked with our pediatrician asked me to breastfeed, just to show her how we were faring. She asked outright about the pain. She listened to my complaints. She told me they were perfectly normal. "It'll get better," she said, "but call anytime. Just to rant."

(And I did: twice, maybe three times. What a gift that was.)

Then, when Alec was maybe six weeks old—by which time we finally had it down to a science, this mammary duet—I took a peek at his growth chart. To my dismay, I saw that his weight had begun to dip below the black curve that marked the "norm" on the graph. When I demanded to know what this meant, the nurse practitioner told me something that shocked me: Here we were in the latter half of the 1990s, yet the standard-issue growth charts still reflected the way babies grow when they're drinking formula—meaning that, to pediatricians ignorant of the difference, breastfed babies did not appear to be growing fast enough. And if formula made a mother's life easier, well, how bad could it be?

Maybe you were told that the pain lasts "only a week or so." Doesn't sound too bad, right? Except that a single week in which you get no more than two or three hours of sleep per night, and in which your waking hours are filled with new and difficult work, seems more like a month . . . especially when your lower torso feels like it's been through the heavyweight championship—against Mike Tyson. How well I remember, the first time around, going through the convoluted ritual (often while Alec cried) of getting my inflatable hemorrhoid doughnut in the just-right spot on the couch, making sure the glass of water and the cushions I needed to buttress the baby were all close at hand, sitting down oh-so-delicately, getting my writhing son in position, hiking up my shirt and bra . . . and then taking a deep, wincing breath as I attached that darling little Hoover to my overworked, traumatized nipple.

"The pain, that's one thing they don't tell you about," says my favorite supermom. "But the other is the time. Because when you nurse, for a while *that's all you do*."

It begins to feel like that movie *Groundhog Day*. You are Bill Murray, minus a good night's sleep; that Sonny and Cher song he has to wake up to, every single day, no end in sight, is the heat-seeking missile of your child's mouth. (Isn't the song in the movie "I Got You Babe"?) Night after night you wake up to those plaintive sobs. Yet again, the digital clock reads 2:53 or 3:02 or maybe even 3:33 exactly. Who says newborns have no sense of time?

Your husband snores blissfully beside you, the light of dawn feels a century distant, and you think, Wait. Didn't this voracious creature—yes, you love him more than anything, you really do!—but didn't he plead starvation an hour ago, an hour before that, and so on? Yet there you are, exhausted to the point of nihilistic despair, trying to summon up the Kama Sutra–like catalog of nursing positions that, if you were lucky, someone in the hospital showed you (while you were zonked on Percocet and the baby was sleeping off the ordeal of birth). Unless you're a saint, the synthetic alternative looks like a million bucks.

My birth instructor said this about nursing: The breast is like a muscle you haven't used yet. "Remember taking up a new sport?" she asked all the earnest young couples in the room. "Remember how the new set of muscles you used surprised you by aching so much?" Well, she said, that's what it's like to use your breasts, the very first time, for the purpose they have been awaiting all your life. "The first few times you do this, they'll ache a bit," she said. "But it's a good kind of ache."

"Ache"? Maybe it's just because I'm a writer and I like the proverbial mot juste, but that mot was so far from juste, it's almost funny. Wasn't "scream in agony" part of her vocabulary? I'd have been happy with "hurt like the dickens." (Did I compare my son's mouth with a vacuum cleaner a page or so back? I meant nail gun.)

Actually, it doesn't hurt so terribly much the first few times—which happen to be the times while you're in the hospital, when "lactation consultants" stop by on a regular basis. The real pain begins when you've been home a couple of days, when your breasts say, "Right, then, time for a break now!"

On one of the first days I ventured out to the grocery store with Alec, two women stopped to admire this brand-new baby. They had young children themselves. One of them asked me how it was going, the nursing part. I knew right away she understood. I said, "God, it hurts! I feel like I've got a humongous paper cut where my nipple used to be." By this time I had tried the ointment mentioned in one book as a remedy for the "abrasion" (the euphemisms never stopped coming). This goo had the tactile appeal of rubber cement and smelled like the sheep barn on my grandparents' farm. And it didn't do much to help me.

One of the women walked over to the produce section and came back with two things: a bunch of carrots and a head of red cabbage, both organic. "Take your pick. Put some in the blender and make a paste," she said. "Hold it on your nipple for fifteen minutes with a wet paper towel, then rinse."

The other woman nodded. "I could tell you're in pain from the way you're walking. That don't-let-my-nipples-touch-my-shirt look."

The Yankee in me was mortified, but the desperate New York mom was touched. I asked these veterans, "Did anyone tell you it would hurt like this?" Both women laughed knowingly. (This laughter was becoming a pattern. Like, why is this such a big secret?) I thanked them, bought the vegetables, went home, and followed their instructions. The paste was soothing—well, a little. My working nipple turned a permanent shade of magenta.

Alec was born during one of the toughest winters I can recall: Snowfall in New York broke all records that year. So mostly we stayed in. The days were long and often lonely; Dennis, Alec's dad, worked till all hours, to make as much money as he could. I went back to my own work, proofreading and editing at home, fitting in as much as Alec's yearnings would allow. I craved human voices, and I craved entertainment. At night, before Dennis got home, I rented all the costume dramas and girl movies he'd never have agreed to watch.

And then, once I managed to cast aside the hemorrhoid doughnut, I discovered how to read a book while nursing. This was a breakthrough. Alec and I had found our favorite daytime position: His belly against mine, he lay on a slight incline, his tiny feet against my right hip. If I put a small, slim cushion on his hip, I could balance a hardcover book on the cushion. Securing him against my body with my right arm, I learned to turn pages with my left.

At first, I felt guilty that I wasn't concentrating on "bonding" with Alec, that I was using him as a lectern of sorts. But right about then, the pain began to fade. Alec was probably three weeks old, though I felt as if I'd known him for that many months. One day I looked down and saw that he'd fallen asleep and away from my breast. I'd been so absorbed in a good novel that I hadn't noticed. Alec's tiny swollen lips still nursed on thin air; my milk lay spilled across his cheek like a sheen of sugar icing. One of his hands still claimed my breast, while his other arm was flung aloft on the pillow, as if he were a cowboy roping a calf. I laid aside my book and just stared. I laughed. *Here it is,* I thought with a sense of wonder and enormous relief. *The bliss.*

I had made it over the hump, no thanks to all the soft-pedalers, the euphemizers, the people I'd relied upon, during my pregnancy, to tell me the unvarnished, apolitical truth about everything. Was that so much to ask? Who thought we weren't tough enough to take it? I knew—unlike my friends who'd done this thing before me—that I was no exception, no freak, no sissy.

My breasts were quite a spectacle. The nursing breast was big, loose, and bawdy, a showgirl gone to seed. The right one, meanwhile, seemed to have shrunk as much as its companion had grown. I was so lopsided that I had begun to develop sciatica on one side (for which I was prescribed a set of exercises, one more thing to fit between Alec's demands).

One night, when I was standing in the bathroom, naked,

Dennis looked at me and smiled mischievously. "Buffy and Lil," he said.

"What?" I said.

"Their names, of course."

I looked in the mirror. I laughed so hard, I had to sit down. That's exactly what they looked like, my breasts: The party girl and the spinster. Mae West and Maggie Smith. Buffy 'n' Lil.

After that, Dennis would come home and ask after them by name.

"How's Buffy holding up today?"

"Hang in there, Lil; wouldn't want you to feel left out."

A few months later, we stayed with friends for a weekend. The first night, after I'd nursed Alec to sleep, I joined three other women in the kitchen, thrilled at the upcoming two or three hours of freedom, freedom to have a meal with grownups, to talk and laugh around a candlelit table, no one appended to me. As it happened, none of my female companions were mothers. One of them asked about nursing, what it was like, and out came the whole grisly tale—with, of course, its happy ending.

"So, are your breasts really huge now?" one woman wanted to know. It was the exuberant hour, the second glass of wine poured, the kitchen filled with scents of a feast: onions, butter, meat, and cake.

"Wanna see?" I said. I pulled up my shirt. "Girls, meet Buffy and Lil."

I heard a round of gasps. "Holy shit," said the woman who'd asked how big they were. When I put down my shirt, we all laughed together.

Ten years later, I remain quite asymmetrical: Lil is as retiring as ever. Buffy's lost much of her moxie, but she's still the star. Sometimes, at the sight of a nursing mother, she sends forth a wishful tingling, just for a moment. Or it might happen while I'm sitting in my office, gazing absently at my books, and I catch sight of a title—*Spartina, A Stone Boat, Dancing After Hours*—one of the many books I read while nursing my two sons. They deserve rereading, these books, because I read them in a mental fog; I did their authors little justice. But when I read them, I was happy. I'd made it up a mountain, and the view was sublime.

❋

Julia Glass is the author of the novels *Three Junes*, which won the 2002 National Book Award for Fiction, and *The Whole World Over*. Her most recent work of fiction is *I See You Everywhere*. She lives in Massachusetts with her family.

FIRST LOVE

Ann Matturro Gault

The words stung at first. I don't know why I needed to know, but at the time it seemed important. "Do you love her more than me?"

He hesitated for a moment, then admitted the truth—"Yes."

Honest to a fault, some would say, but in the fifteen years I've known my husband I've come to accept—no, respect—this about him. Willie is completely sincere. He doesn't sugarcoat anything. And yes, the truth can sometimes hurt, but I still love the guy to pieces. In my experience, working through hard feelings is necessary for real intimacy.

Our engagement in 1995 was a whirlwind. In just ten weeks I planned a December wedding in Midtown that didn't break our bank—or my parents'. My mother suspected our secret but never asked, so we kept it to ourselves. Privately, we were thrilled about my pregnancy. Being unplanned, it had to be a sign that our marriage was meant to be. When I walked down the aisle, only Willie knew I wasn't alone. The baby that would make us a family was along for the ride. When we returned from our honeymoon, we told our parents they'd be grandparents in the spring. (Mom was hurt I'd kept the truth from her, but that's another essay.)

Motherhood didn't intimidate me in the least. I adored babies—especially snuggly newborns—and planned to have a large family. Four or five babies at least. (What can I say? I watched a lot of *The Brady Bunch* while growing up!) Burping, changing, and caring for children seemed to come naturally to me, and I enjoyed caring for my four godchildren. My thickening waist was a happy reminder that at the age of thirty-two I was finally on my way to realizing a long-held dream.

In spite of my eager anticipation, though, I worried about the effect that parenthood would have on my marriage. Since many of my close friends had started their families, I was around babies frequently. I'd witnessed plenty of bickering over whose turn it was to change the poopy diaper and remembered well my own parents' knockdown, dragout fights concerning their three daughters. But Willie and I promised each other to make passion a priority. We wouldn't become mere partners in child care, as so many of our friends had done.

The day after my due date the cramping started, and on the subway ride home from work I had my first full-fledged contraction. Willie came home, and, like the dutiful Lamaze graduates we were, we started to time my contractions. They were irregular—ten minutes, then fifteen, then six minutes apart—but never any closer (it turned out fibroids were to blame). Since they didn't progress in the usual manner, I decided to wait until morning to call the doc. With my husband snoring loudly beside me, I endured the longest night of my life. As soon as daylight hit, I phoned the doctor.

Much, much later that day (around 6:30 P.M.) our little surprise finally arrived. It took thirty-six hours of labor, an episiotomy, and forceps to bring Ryan into the world. She had big blue eyes and the loudest cry in the nursery. My obstetrician, a seasoned pro named Michael O'Leary, was widely regarded as the Forceps Master at New York University Hospital, so when word got out that he would be using them on me, medical students crowded the delivery room. Ryan would arrive in front of a live audience. My husband cut the cord (totally cool for a country boy who grew up hunting deer in his backyard) and took photos of the placenta (this really grossed me out, but he wanted to document the *whole* experience). There were ten fingers and ten toes. All seemed right with the world, and then my milk came in . . .

Nursing got off to a rocky start (with painfully engorged breasts and a sleepy baby as the culprits), but a good book and an unforgettable nurse named Anastasia coached me through it. (Note to expectant mothers: Read *The Nursing Mother's Companion*, by Kathleen Huggins. It should be required reading for anyone planning to breastfeed.)

During my hospital stay I experienced many surprising emotions—hostility, disappointment, and desperation among them. I wanted nursing to come naturally (it didn't). I wanted my husband to fix everything (he couldn't). I'd been so confident that caring for my baby would be easy for a baby whisperer like me. Instead I was throwing myself a full-fledged pity party. Then Dr. O'Leary reminded me who was boss. "Don't let this baby control your life," he warned. "You're the one in charge." Staring down at my beautiful daughter sleeping contentedly in her bassinet (instead of nursing!) made me angry. My boobs hurt and needed emptying. Ryan, still groggy from my epidural, wouldn't wake up. Willie and I tried all the usual tricks—tickling her feet, undressing her, applying a cold washcloth to her forehead—but all she wanted was sleep. As I prayed for her to wake up and eat, it occurred to me that I had never been more out of control in my life—and she wasn't even a week old!

Anastasia assured me that the first two weeks were the hardest, so I figured Ryan and I could tough it out a little longer. Willie was supportive, but there wasn't much he could do aside from bringing me bags of frozen peas and cold cabbage leaves to soothe my aching breasts. He didn't care how I fed our daughter—breast or bottle, the decision was mine.

The convenience of nursing was the initial appeal. I just couldn't see myself mixing, warming, and washing bottles multiple times a day when Mother Nature delivered the milk good to go. In the hospital I learned something else wonderful about breast milk. According to Anastasia, it's the source of that unmistakable newborn smell. So powdery and light, it made me think of angels and permeated everything—even me. My husband lingered a little longer when he hugged me because I, too, had the "baby smell," as we called it. I'd often bury my nose in the chubby folds of Ryan's neck and enjoy a long, intoxicating whiff of the sweet perfume. I concluded it was heaven's scent and that angels were actually babies waiting their turn to be born.

It took a few weeks of practice, but Ryan and I eventually worked out breastfeeding. Ryan turned out to be a good little nurser, and a pattern was soon established. I felt guilty about the negative feelings I'd had at the start. Forgiving my baby— and myself—was the beginning of our bond. Like two girlfriends, we went everywhere together. Since nursing in public never bothered me (yes, it's possible to nurse discreetly), I found Ryan extremely portable. We took long strolls in the park, lunched with friends, and traveled by subway from our new neighborhood in Brooklyn back to my old one in Manhattan. Ryan became well acquainted with the dressing room at Macy's, since nursing melted the baby weight right off me. Less than three months after delivery, new clothes were already in order. I'd lost all of my baby weight (thirty-five pounds) and more. Eating ice cream (my favorite food) as often as I liked didn't take any getting used to. But the best part? I was thin for the first time in my life!

The connection between us was undeniable. My ability to comfort my baby just by offering her the breast astounded me, and Willie was equally impressed. He talked of the power of the dairy bar and even demonstrated it to his friends. When Ryan was about six months old, we attended a party with some of my husband's college friends—many still single at the time. Willie was showing off his daughter when she started to fuss. With baby antennae extended, I approached the group in time to hear him say, "Watch this." Right on cue, Ryan stopped crying the moment he handed her to me.

Poor Daddy; I'm sure he felt like an outsider, but he didn't complain. He'd never have my intimate knowledge of our daughter—God's reward, perhaps, for the hard work of motherhood. He tried to be involved, but nursing was so easy for us that I rarely suggested he give her a bottle. He did come up with a funny little test to determine if Ryan was ready to nurse. Like a human pacifier, he'd insert his finger or the tip of his nose into her mouth. If she started to suck, he knew she was hungry. Of course, I knew when it was feeding time, but I let him enjoy this harmless little ritual.

The milestones during that first year were exciting but bittersweet, too. At four months Ryan discovered her hands, and I loved the way her fat little fingers grabbed at my shirt as she nursed. When she was five months old, I just couldn't get enough of the adorable cooing sounds she made when I came into view (we have a videotape of her doing it). Before long she was enjoying a variety of solid foods. Willie was wild for his little girl and clearly loved feeding her with a spoon. He made up corny little songs as he fed her and obsessively kept her face clean, gently dabbing away excess food with a damp paper towel after every bite. As much as I loved watching the two of them interact, part of me hated sharing her.

At nine months old, Ryan started walking. About the same time (as the pediatrician predicted), she started losing interest in the breast. With all the new places to go, Ryan was just too busy exploring to take time out to nurse. Sadly, I knew this was the first of many steps she would take away from me into her future.

Happily, it wouldn't be long before I'd be given another opportunity to share this special closeness again. I was newly pregnant—with a son—and would go on to have two more daughters afterwards.

Looking back, I know it was breastfeeding that transformed me into a mother. Nursing was our private conversation. Without the exchange of a single word, I always knew what Ryan needed and could easily decipher a hungry cry from a tired one. For the first time in my life, I felt truly important. Some mothers find that dependency suffocating. I cherished it.

The last year had been a whirlwind. Reflecting on all the major transitions made my head spin. I was newly married, I lived in a new neighborhood, and I was a new mother, too. My life had totally changed. The one constant through it all had been my husband. His life was different, but not much. More pressured in his role as provider, perhaps, but he got up in the morning and went to work as usual. Being able to focus on the baby while he took care of the rest was a huge relief to me.

One big thing was different for Willie. He was getting to know his daughter and falling head over heels in love with her. Watching him do this, I saw a tenderness in him that I hadn't seen before. And I fell in love with him again, in a whole new way.

The love for a child feels different from the love for a spouse. More poignant. More intense. And why wouldn't it? Children share your blood, your genes, and, of course, your heart. Willie says he loves Ryan more than me, and though the announcement came as a shock, I'm okay with it now. I've experienced so many firsts with our daughter that I don't mind being number two for now. I was Ryan's first love, after all. When Ryan was born she didn't replace her daddy in my heart. I simply grew another one. Just for her. Only a mother can do that.

※

Ann Matturro Gault spent a decade on the staff of *Family Circle* magazine and now freelances full time. She has written about parenting, health, and education for many publications, including *Redbook*, *Reader's Digest*, *First for Women*, and Scholastic.com. Gault lives with her husband and their four children in New Jersey.

ANTI-DEPRESSED MILK

Rebecca Walker

I knew I would breastfeed almost immediately after my mother told me that while she nursed me, I had bitten her nipple so hard it started to bleed. She didn't tell me this with malice; she experienced pain, and I was, objectively, the cause of that pain. Nonetheless, when she told me, and every time I thought of it after, I felt a hideous conflagration of emotions. Shame, anger, disbelief—they all coursed through me as I wondered what sort of infant would do such a horrible thing.

I was twelve years old when my mother told me what I had done to her. An image formed instantly: my mother's faultless nipple, raw and bloody, my own teeth marks around the areola. I never looked at a breast in the same way again. I began to have dreams that my own breasts were being cut, mutilated, torn to bits. With a child's logic, I decided that when the time came I would breastfeed successfully; I would not put my child or myself through such agony.

It hurts to remember these things, to have to revisit the imagined ripping of my tender, defenseless breasts. But it must be done. Otherwise, it would be impossible to understand why, after I had my son and nursed him for the first time in the neonatal intensive care unit where he was strapped to a board before I could reach him, I felt my breasts miraculously restored to their full, uncut selves. As he sucked hungrily and I offered copiously, I wept silent, grateful tears. My breasts had not been destroyed. My son, though ill, was alive.

The nurses seemed to understand the miraculous healing of my wounds. After that first day, they called me with their singsong voices from the Philippines, Guyana, and Brooklyn. Mommy Walker, they would yell, your baby is hungry! And I would bolt out of bed and throw on the gray robe I had impulsively bought at a maternity shop weeks before. I would make my way to the ICU, where I could hear my son's screams yards before I reached the locked door.

The nurses would buzz me in and organize Tenzin's monitor leads while I washed and dried my hands. There was the lead that measured how much oxygen was in Tenzin's blood; there was the one that monitored how fast his heart was beating. There was the oxygen tube that had to remain in place at all times, but in such a way that his face could still be pressed against my breast. There was the careful placement of my baby into my arms.

They did all of this, and then they brought me water, too, and I never saw them do that for the other mothers. They put a stool beneath my feet, too, one that I never saw in the ICU when my feet weren't resting on it. They stroked my hair and patted my hand. They told me that many babies had meconium aspiration syndrome, that it was not so bad. Then they showed me, again, how I should hold Tenzin so that he could get a good latch. So that he would be able to get from me what he needed in order to live and be strong.

We had a honeymoon of sorts, my son and I, but then, rain. My son was not growing, and while breastfeeding was cathartic for me, it seemed to be causing Tenzin some difficulty. Because I had so much milk, a kind of geyser-like overflow, I might be overwhelming or, as one nurse offered, "drowning" my son with it. When Tenzin tried to breathe and also to suck, he found it almost impossible to do both; he could not coordinate his breathing with his sucking. At a certain point the question was put to me: Which did he need more, to breastfeed or to breathe?

It seems obvious, but when asked the question I could not immediately see the answer. I felt that his drinking milk from my breast was as essential as his being fed through our shared umbilical cord. The idea of cutting this connection (again!) was too shocking. We had just found each other! My breasts were just beginning to heal after decades! Tenzin spent most of his hours inside a medical crib in a locked and sterile unit; surely we could not also deprive him of my breasts! At some point the doctor ordered, matter-of-factly, that I pump and bottle-feed.

I was devastated. That evening my husband came to my room—*our* room by this point, as I had hung huge paintings of Buddhas all over the dingy walls and had an iPod playing ragas, Björk, and Gil Scott-Heron constantly, and we had stocked a huge cooler with organic food and bottles of water. He strode in, tall and strong, and said that the doctor had mentioned bottle feeding to him. I burst into tears. I can't let go of breastfeeding, I said. Tenzin needs me to breastfeed. He mustn't grow up without that bond. We lost our first moments together. I cannot lose this. My breasts ached. Out of the corner of my eye I could see the yellow pump the nurse had rolled in a few hours before.

This is about the baby, my husband said. Then he held me in his arms and let me cry for a long time. I know, he said. I know this is hard. And he also said, Pumping and giving the baby a bottle is the best thing to do. And I nodded, because I could remember that morning, when I had tried to feed Tenzin, and he looked as if he couldn't breathe but the milk was flooding into his mouth anyway.

I began to pump. I put suction cups in a special bra that held them in place while the machine pulled the milk out of me. It is a cliché, I know, but I felt like a cow. I was not altogether unhappy about being milked by the machine, but I did feel like a cow. I also felt, while I was sitting in my hospital room and my baby was in the ICU with oxygen tubes in his nose, that at least I was doing something, I was *pumping*, and that was quite a bit. And it was literally quite a bit, quite a lot, actually, so much that whenever I strolled into the ICU, looking self-satisfied with three or more full bottles in my hand for the refrigerator, the nurses would turn to me and ask, You have more? We need a whole fridge just for Mommy Walker's milk! And I would, finally, grin like an Olympic athlete who has just won the gold.

It was, again, a brief respite.

Brief because there was another problem with my breastfeeding, and with my affair with breastfeeding. This was the fact that I was on medication for depression. My breast milk was tainted with that medication, and I lived in California, the land of the pure and organic, and there was some very limited evidence of a correlation between maternal use of this drug and seizures in newborns. I had asked my ob-gyn, my homeopath, my Tibetan doctor, experts from at least three dozen sites on the Internet, and then, finally, the nursing consultant in the hospital if there was a risk of hurting my baby with my anti-depressed milk. They had all said no, and I believed exactly none of them.

In fact, I had a running tabulation in my mind of my son's exposure to the antidepressants. I had allowed the nine months of exposure in utero, because if I hadn't I might have awaked one morning so depressed I couldn't remember why I was having a baby in the first place. After the birth, whether to continue the drug, to continue nursing, or both was up for negotiation. Oh, how I wanted to give my baby the gift of twelve months of breast milk! Oh, how I knew I couldn't live with myself if I gave in to that longing! I knew I could, in good conscience, nurse for three months, maybe even five. Tenzin's cells will grow fat with my milk, I thought, and then we can switch to organic formula.

In the end, my son drank breast milk for three and a half months. He drank it plentifully from the bottle in the hospital, and once he could breathe on his own he drank from my breasts. He grew, in those three months and every month thereafter, into the happiest and healthiest of babies.

I had wanted an uncomplicated bond with my son. He would not bite my nipple off, he would not wound me irreparably, he would not cause me to reject him and spend the rest of his life feeling a queer kind of guilt. No. He would be the beneficiary of all the work I had done on myself: work to get the image of my breasts being cut off out of my head, work to keep my depression at bay so I wouldn't kill anyone or myself, work to find a mate and love a mate and let a mate love me.

In my fantasy my son would not be sick, and we would nurse every day bathed in a beautiful soft light. I would rock him in a rocker and I would love him and he would love me and the sum total of all of that would be that he would go to a good college and be a successful human being and all of my perfect parenting would, in fact, mean that I would never die.

It wasn't until I returned home from living at the hospital for a month that I began to separate reality from my wild imaginings. I came to realize that certain things would happen. My son would live, and I would be less depressed, and my husband would love me. I knew I would eventually feed my son formula, and he would still love me, and still need me, and I would still love him and still need him. I would come to see that it isn't about the breasts at all, this powerful love between mother and child.

Or at least, as I came to find out, it doesn't have to be.

❋

Rebecca Walker is an award-winning, best-selling author and speaker whose books include *To Be Real: Telling the Truth and Changing the Face of Feminism*; *Black, White, and Jewish: Autobiography of a Shifting Self*; and *Baby Love: Choosing Motherhood after a Lifetime of Ambivalence*.

DOUBLE TROUBLE

Suzanne Schlosberg

I used to think that the most boring person alive was Steve Forbes, the former Republican presidential candidate who droned on for a decade about replacing the federal income tax with a 17 percent flat tax on personal and corporate earnings.

But I was wrong. It's not Steve Forbes. It's me. Because all I talk about these days is breastfeeding.

Consider: Last week at the supermarket I ran into an elderly couple from the neighborhood. Though we ostensibly had plenty to chat about—their trip to Florida, our town's new Thai restaurant—somehow, within seconds, I turned the conversation to my milk supply. Marlene managed to feign interest, but poor Nathan was reduced to reading the nutrition labels on the ground beef.

Worse: Last weekend at a bat mitzvah party, the president of our synagogue's board of directors marched over, grabbed my hand, and said, "Could you stop talking about breastfeeding for five minutes and come dance?"

But what's there not to talk about? Feeding my four-month-old twin boys is the driving force of my existence. In my every waking moment, I'm never more than two and a half hours from the next nursing or pumping session, which means if I'm not nursing or pumping, then I'm thinking about the next time I have to nurse or pump and calculating how to squeeze the rest of my life into the window between. My breastfeeding schedule dictates everything, even down to where I get my snow tires installed. (Every year it's been Costco, where I brave the long lines in exchange for the low cost. But this year I paid double at a local garage because the wait at Costco would have been longer than my breasts could withstand.)

The other day a friend startled me with this question: "What do you like most about motherhood?" She might as well have asked, "What do you like most about Slovenia?" The thing is, I don't really think of myself as a mother. I think of myself as a breastfeeder.

It's true that I'm the one who delivered my twins—one vaginally and the other via c-section, which, technically, makes me not only a mother but also a war hero. And yet I feel I've done so little mothering. I would venture to say that my husband, who bathes the boys before bed and massages them with lotion while I work in my office, does the bulk of the mothering. Even when I'm singing "The Wheels on the Bus" to the boys on the morning shift, my mind is wandering: How much will I be able to accomplish before the next feeding?

A friend suggested that my preoccupation with breastfeeding is biologically driven—that new mothers are programmed to be so single-minded because otherwise their babies would starve. It's a good point. I'm acutely aware that a few wrong moves—a couple of mistimed dermatologist's appointments or a six-hour wait at Costco—and my milk supply will dry up like Lake Anguli Nur in China.

Before the boys were born, I wouldn't have pegged myself as the type to blather on about nursing. After all, when I was pregnant I rarely talked about my pregnancy. What was there to say? I was fat. I had heartburn. My ankles were swollen. None of this struck me as newsworthy. Pregnancy was easy to dismiss as a conversation topic because, other than monthly doctor's visits and a trip to the jeweler to get my wedding ring sawed off, it required nothing of me. I was pregnant the same way I was left-handed: I just was. But breastfeeding is different, not only because it demands so much of my attention but also because my milk supply has been so hard-earned.

Toby and Ian were born a month early, weighing about five pounds each, with less body fat than Nicole Richie pre-rehab and even less interest in sucking. When presented with my nipples, they were at a complete loss, as if someone had offered them fly-fishing rods. They'd fall asleep or cry or flail about, but rarely would they suck. Without sufficient stimulation, I was producing no milk. The hospital outfitted me with an industrial-grade breast pump that looked like it could extract breast milk from my deceased grandmothers, and I dutifully cranked it every three hours, twenty-four hours a day.

But still, no milk.

To help the boys along, the nurses hooked us up with a remedial nursing system, training wheels for the lactationally challenged. Clipped to each of my bra straps were small, formula-filled bottles with tiny hoses dangling from them. I'd tape the hoses to my breasts, then insert the ends into the corner of the boys' mouths. The idea was that the babies would think they were breastfeeding when, in fact, they were sucking formula through a straw. My boys did not seem to appreciate the leg up and would expend huge amounts of energy shrieking and yanking the tubes off my breasts.

All of this was monumentally distressing. I couldn't help but feel that I was failing Toby and Ian. (I'll admit that, at a low point, I tried to get them to shoulder some of the blame and blurted out, "You people have only one job—to suck—and you can't even do that?" I later apologized.)

After four days in the hospital our problem moved home, along with all my anxieties. The situation remained so frustrating and so utterly ridiculous that my breastfeeding, or lack of it, was unquestionably my biggest headline when my friends asked how I was doing. And they seemed rapt as I described our strategies to keep the boys from falling asleep on the job, like tugging at their ears, tickling their feet, and promising to buy them video games when they grew up, the kinds with Uzis, suicidal terrorists, and mutilated female corpses.

We abandoned the hose system—you can't use training wheels forever—and, gradually, the boys did start to catch on, though not enough to earn any Boy Scout badges. Toby would lick instead of suck. "It's a nipple," I'd plead, "not an ice-cream cone." Ian would spit out my nipple fifteen or twenty times per feeding, as if he were being force-fed Brussels sprouts.

I'm certain I'd have thrown in the towel if not for the encouragement of a friend with twins who had persevered through ten weeks of the same problems, plus a breast infection and cracked and bleeding nipples. I felt like a demoralized marathon runner who's on the verge of dropping out of the race—until someone with an artificial leg hobbles by. Quitting was not an option.

Plus, mercifully, there was Charlotte. Charlotte was our baby nurse, generously underwritten by my parents for our first two weeks of parenthood and imported from Los Angeles, where they live, because there was no such person as a baby nurse in my town. (I live in Do-It-Yourselferville, and though I'd like to maintain the delusion that I could have done it myself, I'm skeptical, and utterly grateful I didn't have to find out.)

I adored Charlotte, mostly because she was even less domestic than me. Charlotte was incapable of loading a dishwasher—she'd arrange five dishes and suddenly the dishwasher was full—and her scrambled eggs were both burned and runny, if that's even possible. This was a woman who had raised three children. There was hope for me, after all.

Charlotte was intimately involved in our fledgling breast-feeding operation. Every three hours, she'd bring the boys to me in bed and then stand by my side and knead my breasts, imploring them to produce more milk and cheering on the boys as they thrashed around in the vicinity of my nipples. After my ten minutes of quasi nursing, Charlotte would bottle-feed one baby with a mixture of formula and breast milk while my husband bottle-fed the other, and I would pump. We made for a great threesome. I was sad to see Charlotte go.

Charlotte's replacement, Sally, a grandmother of eight, billed herself as a doula—available "to do whatever a mother needs," according to her resumé—but seemed to have a single goal: to do as little as possible. Upon arrival, at 11:00 P.M., she would yawn and whine, "Ooooh, I'm soooo tired." (She was tired? One morning I applied mascara under my eyes instead of concealer, accidentally achieving the linebacker look.) Once, at 4:00 A.M., Sally carried the boys into my bedroom and announced, "Okay, they're ready to eat!" when, in fact, the boys were nearly comatose. Clearly, she was trying to unload them so she could go home.

Sally made no attempt to conceal her disapproval of our breast-bottle-pump triumvirate. She inspected my nipples, pronounced them "marvelous," and insisted that if only I took vitamin B_{12} complex, my breasts would flow like the Trevi Fountain. (I did take vitamin B_{12} complex, plus various herbs and teas, and none of it made a difference.) Sally lasted three days.

After six weeks of audacious effort, my milk was finally flowing. The boys were nursing like champs, and I could handle the whole operation solo. Breastfeeding became such a nonevent that I could manage it while reading a magazine— a feat that, early on, seemed as improbable as my learning to juggle while riding a unicycle.

But even though the big headlines have vanished, my obsession has remained. Whereas previously I was consumed with my shortcomings, now I'm completely caught up in the complexities of this whole process. Take, for instance, how I've mastered breastfeeding two babies at the same time.

Tandem nursing is not something you do at Starbucks. I see women breastfeeding while chatting with friends and sipping a latte and marvel at how discreetly it can be done. Tandem nursing is more like a piece of performance art involving a bed, numerous props, and, inevitably, exposed breasts. There's no stylish shawl that can shield the public from the spectacle of two four-month-olds sucking down their lunch. You'd have to erect a four-person tent.

These days I nurse my boys on a twin bed in their room. I place one Boppy pillow on each end of the bed, then plant one baby on each Boppy while I buckle myself into a giant, U-shaped foam pillow that my friend Sarah has dubbed the "life raft," all the while asking my wailing boys to forgive me for the delay. I place another foam pillow between my back and the

wall, then hoist each baby atop the life raft and shove one
Boppy under each side of it, to make the surface flat so that the
babies don't roll off.

Like I said, not something you do at Starbucks.

Once they get going, I never fail to be impressed with their
competence and to note that each has developed his own signature style. Ian sucks rhythmically, with his eyes closed and
long lashes fluttering, and appears to be concentrating hard, as
if he's doing calculus in his little, lopsided head. Toby operates
entirely on instinct. He sucks erratically, with his plump little
fists planted on his temples, as if to say, "Oy vey, the brisket is
undercooked."

Sometimes, when he's really hungry, he'll . . .

Oh, dear. I'm doing it again. I'm being boring.

When I think about how my life has come to this, I tend to
start counting up all the hours I'm now devoting to breastfeeding. Some babies take five minutes to suck down a meal,
but, perhaps making up for all those weeks of trying, Toby and
Ian prefer to linger at the table. (Lactation consultants call babies like mine "gourmet eaters.") Sometimes I nurse for forty
minutes, not counting the setup time. Multiply that by four,
then add in two half-hour pumping sessions (to produce
enough milk for the boys' daily bottle, given to them by our
babysitter while I work). Then multiply it all by seven, and I'm
spending upwards of twenty-five hours a week simply feeding
my children.

Maybe breastfeeding is all I talk about because, some days,
it's practically all I do.

I know, I know. Breastfeeding is supposed to be a special
time of intimacy and bonding. Well, when I calculate that I've
probably spent as much time breastfeeding in the past four

months as some women spend in a year, I have to wonder: How much more bonding do the three of us really need?

I'm already itching to quit, or at least scale back. I'd like to retrieve some of that time so I can do things that make me feel more like a mother than a breastfeeder. I want to sing "The Wheels on the Bus" without looking at the clock, and I want to know my children better when they're not eating. I'd like for their dad to take over some of the feedings so that, sometimes, I can be the one to pick out their sleepers and toys at Target. And let's deal with reality: I'd like more time so I can earn the money to pay for those sleepers and toys. If I just had a few extra hours, then I think I could put an end to this compulsive need to discuss my milk supply and stop being the most boring person alive.

I know that day will come soon enough, but right now it seems a lifetime away. And so I talk, and I continue to test my friends' patience. When I apologized to one friend last week for prattling on about my noisy breast pump, she cheerily told me I wasn't a bother at all.

"You think you're boring now?" she said. "Wait until all you talk about is potty training."

✳

Suzanne Schlosberg earns her living as both a humorist and a health writer. Among her publications are *The Curse of the Singles Table: A True Story of 1001 Nights without Sex*, *The Essential Fertility Log*, and *The Ultimate Workout Log*. Suzanne lives with her husband and twin sons in Bend, Oregon.

BREAST-LAID PLANS

Heidi Raykeil

"By the way," says the woman clearing the table, "I think it's great—what you're doing . . ." She speaks in a low, conspiratorial voice and nods towards the baby at my breast, but it still takes me a minute to get what she's talking about. "What I'm doing" is openly nursing my six-week-old baby in the middle of a county fair food court. Up to that point it never occurred to me that I might be making someone uncomfortable by nursing; I'm a liberal city girl, and my baby is young enough still to fall into the "appropriate nursing age" category. Yet at that point I realized that among all the women and babies I've seen here strolling about, enjoying the animals and elephant ears and famous scones, I have not seen one other nursing mother.

Nursing this baby I have to be a little more obvious than I like to be. She is having a hard time with her latch, her little head bobs and bounces, and she refuses to open her eyes, flailing at the breast like a newborn puppy. My nipple sticks out, at attention, waiting to be useful. It's frustrating, and hard to be discreet—not that I'm trying to be. I never planned on being an advocate for breastfeeding; I'm more mellow than militant, more shy than showy. And yet I nursed my older daughter until she was three and a half. And yet here I am, letting it all hang out. Here I am, inadvertent activist, feeding my baby among dirty looks and suckling cows and pigs—laughing to myself at the irony in that, and musing how parenthood and planning have so little to do with each other.

The trouble I'm having breastfeeding this baby is another one of those parenting surprises—after all, I'm an expert, right? But tell that to my nipples, sore and raw as the virgin skin I had six and a half years ago, when I struggled with my older daughter the same way. I never planned on breastfeeding her as long as I did. Now, when friends ask why she nursed so long, I usually give the easy answer: She had a hard time latching on, and when she finally got it she didn't want to give it up. But, of course, there is much more to the story than that. When it comes to parenting, isn't there always more?

✳   ✳

While I wait for my husband and six-year-old daughter to come back from their cotton candy and roller coaster adventures, I nurse the baby again, and again we struggle. I bolster myself by making a mental list of all the reasons breastfeeding is important to me, all the reasons I'm willing to put up with the pain and hassle of these early weeks:

I am favored
I am flavored!
the feeling of letting down
oxytocin
setting an example

burning extra calories!

baby gazing

boobs-a-rama

no binkies

no bottles

no period

goopy-eye cute!

milk on tiny lashes

The baby makes another hungry strike at my breast, turning angry and bright red until, suddenly, she's on. Her color goes back to normal, and instantly her body goes limp, falling into me, forming to me, milk-drunk. And it hits me—this is the real reason I love breastfeeding. This moment. It's not something you can put on a list; it's one of life's biologically reinforced, beautiful intangibles. It is the surprise of direct connection, ultimate intimacy, the trust and ability to go back, if even for a fifteen-minute feeding, to a time when two separate beings were one. I also sometimes hate parenting because of this moment: It is so elusive, so private and ephemeral. There is no one clear-cut way to reach it, no how-to book or magic recipe, no amount of planning in the world that can guarantee this outcome.

✳   ✳

The lactation consultant the hospital provided when I had my older daughter was no help to me at all. Her callused hands worked my breasts with the warmth and charm of a dairy farmer until, frustrated, she left the room in a huff, leaving me with her final advice: "Sometimes it just doesn't work out." I cried as she left, then fumed, then laughed cynically with my husband as we made up excuses for her bad behavior: Clearly she was an unhappy person, engorged with a need to spray bad attitude and ruin a new parent's joyous day. And then we calmly finger-fed our daughter and cooed over her in hushed delight. The truth is, we had recently seen another, grimmer version of "doesn't work out" that made my daughter's trouble at the breast seem like a small, surmountable step on the unpredictable precipice of parenting.

I always planned to breastfeed my babies; as a child of hippies, naked babies and naked boobies were the norm. By the time I was pregnant I had heard horror stories of chapped and bleeding nipples, unrelenting mastitis, and other booby blues, but I was sure things would be fine, that things would all go our way, that things would go as planned. Then again, that was before I had kids, back when I knew everything. That was before I had heard the saying "Want to make God laugh? Tell her your plans"—and knew how true it could be.

A year and a half before our older daughter was born, I gave birth to our first child, a beautiful, golden-haired boy named Johnny. Johnny was born with severe, unexplained brain damage. Right after delivery they whisked him away from me. By the time I saw him they had him so hooked up with cords and wires there was no chance for me to hold him at all, much less breastfeed. For twelve days I sat by his small plastic incubator with the devil called helplessness. For twelve days I made the trip down the hall every three hours to the small, quiet milk-pumping room to do the only productive thing I could. In that room, Johnny and I had a whole imagined world of intimacy. In that room, I imagined the giant loud machine was him, sucking at my breast, coming back to me, to where we were one, one painful ounce at a time. Breast milk is the literal expression of hope. This is breastfeeding, for me: what you can give, when you can.

After Johnny died, it took weeks for my milk to dry up. My body was as shocked by the sudden change of plans as my heart; my rock-hard breasts leaked and cried right along with me. "Let me nurture," they seemed to shout, "Let me mother." Losing Johnny was a crash course in mothering, a short, striking lesson in what really matters in life and love and parenting and planning. The minute he was born we let go of all our plans for him and committed ourselves to him as he actually was. And then we had to let go of those plans, too.

Sometimes I think I nursed my daughter so long because, quite simply, I could. But there were other reasons as well. Nursing gave me so much; it got me through that first tough year, through the grief that I was still hot and full and hard with. Breastfeeding my daughter taught me to trust my body again, to feel safe in the world, to count on something and have somebody count on me. When she was an infant, nursing gave my daughter the same sense of trust. When she was a toddler, it gave her the freedom to be independent, by serving as an anchor in the sea of the tumultuous twos. When she was a three-year-old, it gave her something to fall back on as she pushed forward in her expanding world. And all the while it helped me become whole again. It sustained me, and it tethered me with a safe, predictable connection to the most important thing in the world.

❋   ❋

"Mom! You've *got* to see this!" My daughter comes running, her face dirty and sticky with sweets far less natural than the mother's milk she loved so much as a baby. She grabs the baby's pinkie and pulls us both into a stall where fair goers are rapidly gathering. It is yet another surprise: piglets! We ooh and aah together over them, and then suddenly the pen erupts into a shrieking frenzy—feeding time. The piglets fight and jockey for nipples; the crowd standing around watching gets larger and louder. It is a loud, beautiful, chaotic mess. The baby cries from all the noise and I feel my own milk letting down. I work my way over to the corner, where I score a small milking stool to sit on. I lift up my shirt to feed her, and for a moment I worry what everyone will think. By the time the baby is latched on and I finally look up, I'm surprised all over again. Around me I see only kind nods of approval, and I hear gentle laughter from other parents acknowledging the comedy and connection in this moment, acknowledging that we're all in this together, standing tough like that mother pig, giving what we can, when we can, without the protection of a map, a plan, or even a good nipple shield to protect us from the pain.

❊

Heidi Raykeil is the author of *Confessions of a Naughty Mommy: How I Found My Lost Libido*. Her writing has been featured in *Parenting* magazine and online at *Literary Mama*. She lives in Seattle with her family.

NOTHING AT
ALL TO SAY

Deborah Garrison

Again she winds up
to suck, clutched to my belly,
cranking her free arm and cracking
at the breast as though to break me,
the mouth shivering at mere air before it's fit
there: the blunt starburst of pain, pure metal,
cutting me to the core and from somewhere obscure
within comes the tingled press forward of my self,
liquidly, yet concentrated to a single
arrow's point, aimed at the roof of her mouth
and sticking there. She at first jawing in drowning
gasps, noisily, while her hand beats arhythmically,
now more gently slapping the upper shelf of the breast
as though plumping it until the full power flows in—
at which she breaks off, head tossed back,
a pause before surrender,
lips poised in fresh star.
The nipple prinks, sharp-appearing
in this drama of reattachment

at last achieved. At last
drinking steadily, her fingers lightly
twisting in air, lithe and playing at a music,
drifting.
Motes of nothing cross us.
Nothing at all to say or be but this.
Simple like no other thing.
How smoothly then, machine-like
the chik-chikking me-to-her of the pull and release,
the almost chewing, with quickish nosey breaths . . .
After some minutes so faintly the suck is barely
there, but if you tug gently the bud lock trembles and holds,
the draw reasserts, and you float into the drink
with her, now so peaceably twisting
the skin of your forearm. Chik-chik-chik.
Still some milk.
Soon asleep.

※

Deborah Garrison is the author of the poetry collections *The Second Child* and *A Working Girl Can't Win*. She lives with her husband and children in Montclair, New Jersey.

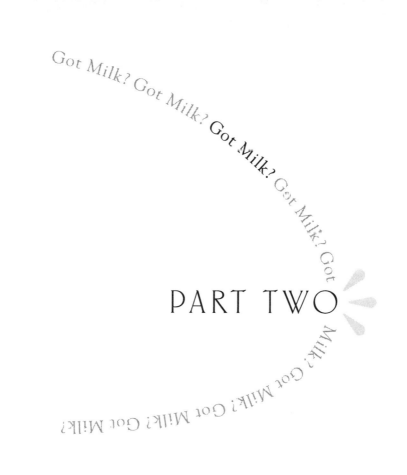

Got Milk? Got Milk? Got Milk? Got Milk? Got Milk? Got Milk? Got Milk? Got Milk? Got Milk?

PART TWO

ONLY THE BABY HAS NOWHERE TO GO

Rachel Zucker

Judah is nursing in his sleep. The weight of his head is pressing uncomfortably against the muscle of my right arm as I write. When his sucking slows down, I jostle him slightly until he sucks harder.

Everyone has a theory of how to make babies sleep better. At four months post partum every theory appeals to me; sleep is so precious and in such short supply. My pediatrician suggested I "top the baby off" with formula because "it has lots of good calories." My stepmother claims her cohort nursed their babies only during the day; at night the babies were fed formula by baby nurses. Grandmothers everywhere tell me to give my baby rice cereal so "he has just a little something in his stomach." But postpartum doulas and lactation advocates say breast-fed babies sleep just as well (which is to say, just as poorly) as formula-fed babies. Breastfeeding advocates view the pressure to start solids or offer formula to lengthen sleep as part of the culture's attempt to dissuade women from breastfeeding. Other than where and how we birth our babies, sleep is the most controversial parenting topic in the first six to twelve months.

What does nursing have to do with sleep? Today is Judah's four-month birthday. He is beautiful and big and happy and a great joy to our family. And I'm tired. So tired. Everything has to do with sleep.

∗   ∗

The first two minutes on this uncomfortable couch with my battery-powered nursing light, notebook, and pen were *brutal*. But I'm okay now. He *did it*. At 2:30 A.M. he squawked for a few minutes and then went back to sleep. Hurrah! It's 4:35 A.M. Oh, he's coughing and sputtering. My let-down is strong, my breasts very full. He keeps pulling off, coughing, then lunging back for the nipple. The early days of nursing were like this—suck, sputter, choke, suck—but this is the exception now rather than the rule.

Usually I nurse him in bed, in the dark, this early in the morning and doze off and on while he nurses. Judah will growl or punch at me, and I'll wake enough to adjust my body so he can latch on.

The early-morning nursing is a vestige of the first three months when we slept together all night, or, more accurately, lay in bed together for many hours in a drowsy, fevered, milky darkness. At three months I started to move Judah to the Co-Sleeper (the small baby bed attached to my bed) or to the crib after each feeding. The change was bittersweet. I could tell he had been sucking to suck, not for milk, and because he was getting milk all night he was nursing less during the day. I had offered him a pacifier or my finger to satisfy his sucking needs, but neither worked. We had been sleeping less and less. I had developed a chronic pain in my shoulder from long hours of nursing while lying on my side.

The same shoulder hurts now. I'm twisted around, trying to write while shielding Judah from the half-covered nursing light. Will I be able to go back to sleep? I'm very awake now.

✝   ✝

I hate pumping! I love the freedom it affords me—I'm going to take my two older sons to school and then write for two hours while my husband stays home with the baby—but I hate pumping! I feel like a cow hooked up to a milking machine. My big boys are fighting, the baby is looking at me longingly, but I can't get up. *Flewp, flewp, flewp,* goes the machine, while I make a speech to the big boys: "Every day is a new day." In other words, Don't tell your brother you won't play with him for three days. Now Moses is amusing the baby—scratch that, now the boys are fighting over who gets to amuse the baby. "You need to get dressed," I say to Abram for the millionth time. The fact that I'm tethered to this machine, which is plugged into the wall, is undermining my authority. "We don't *need* to do anything," says Abram. "Yes, we do *need* to do things," says Moses in his most condescending older-brother voice. Now they're arguing about whether or not they *need* to do anything.

*   *

Judah drank two ounces while I was out. My breasts feel full. I'm so happy to see him and grateful to be released from the pressure of writing. This is the third week of our new writing/child-care schedule. It's still hard for me to leave Judah on the two mornings I take the boys to school and write, and it's overwhelming how carefully organized everything needs to be.

Judah is holding my left hand. Now he's kicking his feet. He's rubbing his eyes. He wants to nurse to sleep, but I'm not going to let him. Just another minute of this sweetness. His body is heavy—he's fussing—sucking hard now . . . He's asleep. Oh, well.

*   *

It's quiet. The baby and I are alone in the apartment. The big boys are with their grandparents; my husband is working. I finished a long poem during Judah's nap. I had to fight the urge to call a friend just now when I saw he wanted to nurse. I won't. I'll just sit on the couch and nurse and write and look at the wrecked living room (toys, clothes, papers everywhere) and do nothing about it. The mess is the result of writing, and I'm proud to have chosen writing over cleaning. Must order groceries. Must make lists. Must remember to write pediatrician appointments into my datebook. Not now; just sit here.

I spaced out for a few minutes. Thinking half thoughts that float by without pressure, like the savasana state of mind that yoga teachers describe and that I usually have trouble achieving.

*   *

I'm so tired of feeling drugged. I'm starting to float. The sensation might not be unpleasant except for the ache in my head. I was falling asleep, waiting to feed him, but writing always wakes me up. In this way writing is the opposite of nursing. While nursing I zone out; writing wakes up my mind, sharpens it. Nursing is soft and fuzzy-minded; it is floaty and loose and diffuse. Writing focuses the mind and magnifies everything around.

A few weeks ago I was complaining about something to my husband while I was nursing. Half-joking and half-serious, my husband said, "Hey, don't give him any of that nervous milk." I wonder if writing while nursing has any effect on either the supply or the quality of milk.

Oops, I sneezed, and Judah startled. Now he is gently scratching at my ribs through my T-shirt. I just want to put my head down and rest.

*   *

Below the half-lowered shade I can see Manhattan. So many lights still on—are all those people feeding babies? Another light comes on across the way. People are watching TV or having sex or playing computer games. They should go to sleep!

This project was to write *while* nursing but not necessarily *about* nursing. Maybe I have nothing else to write about. Nursing. Sleep. Lack of sleep. Is that all I think about? No. I think my friend Nathan should be happier than he is. I think my son Abram believes he has to break a bone to get my attention. I think Bush sucks. I think too much of motherhood is about withstanding physical discomfort.

*   *

Pumping. I'm running late this morning. Feel hung-over but no time for a shower. The milk is not coming out. I focus on my let-down, imagine the look and feel of the baby nursing. That's better. Here it comes. The slurp of the Pump In Style (stupid name), my oldest son whistling, my middle son asking, "Do I *have* to wear these pants?" and my husband: "I asked you to clean this up!" The milk looks thin and watery. We all have what storyteller Dovie Thomason calls "hurry-up sickness." Only the baby has nowhere to go and nothing to do. "Well, clean up *later*; now you've got to come and eat breakfast!" roars my husband. The baby is practicing rolling from side to side and back. My husband comes out and clucks at the baby, raspberries him. "Is this your *friend?*" he asks, holding a toy elephant in front of the baby, his high, musical voice so different from the voice he uses with the two big boys.

* *

Everything feels like too much today. I'm working on my poetry when I'm not with the baby, writing in the nursing notebook when I'm nursing, and trying to do everything else— minding the boys, food shopping and preparation, answering emails, cleaning, keeping up with friends, spending time with my husband—when the baby is asleep or copacetic. I'm frazzled. Maybe keeping the nursing journal is just too much. Maybe I need the do-nothingness of nursing. Maybe the zoning out of the nursing mind is restorative the way rapid-eye-movement sleep is. I remember reading that scientists can't figure out exactly how sleep works, even though the disastrous effects of sleep deprivation are well documented. We don't know why, but we need to sleep.

* *

On the M11 bus, going to pick up the boys. I took a two-and-a-half-hour nap during the baby's three-hour (!) nap. Felt wild, weird, and hungry when I woke up. Much better, though—not angry, not toxic.

I'm standing up in the crowded bus and nursing Judah in the Ergo sling. My breast is partially exposed, but no one in this crowd cares. An overweight woman is taking up three seats at the front of the bus. "What the fuck are you staring at, Dirt Boy?" she yells at someone. The baby pulls off to look her way, and I slide my shirt down over my nipple.

* *

On the bus home with the boys. They're thumb wrestling. The boy behind me is kicking my seat. The baby is whining. There's so much stimulation: rustling bags, noisy kids, the bus's engine, the fried-chicken smell of KFC. The baby is sucking his way into privacy and comfort, but from my perspective the sucking is another imposition. It feels invasive. Ouch! He keeps clamping down on my nipple and turning his head towards various distractions without letting go. Meanwhile, a nanny is giving me dirty looks—why? Oh, for scribbling in my notebook while my big boys push each other.

* *

Lying in bed. The city is misty and gray. Judah rests his foot on my belly. His toes are curled like a baby monkey's. I'm leaking from the breast he's not sucking; a dark circle is growing larger on my T-shirt. We're animals now. His hair is sweaty from the hard work of a long sleep. I'm still unshowered and smell like sweat, breast milk, spit-up, and baby pee.

Judah pulls off, flashes me a drunken smile, pats my still-soft stomach, and goes back to business.

This is the room in which he was born. Right there, in a birthing tub, at the foot of the bed. We lay here, in this bed, together, the whole family, right after I delivered the placenta, and the baby nursed his first long nurse. We were animals then, too. Beautiful animals.

*   *

Talking to my husband.

*   *

Watching *Weeds* with my husband.

*   *

In line at the post office to mail my new manuscript.

*   *

In the hallway of the school.

*   *

Back home for a proper, sit-down nursing. P.U.! The baby is so gassy! What did I eat today?

The big boys are arguing in the other room.

*   *

Helping with homework.

✳   ✳

Supervising violin practice.

✳   ✳

Just woke Judah from a late nap; he's none too pleased. Dinner was unexpectedly momentous. We hadn't planned on it, but we ended up explaining sex to the boys. They know so much about pregnancy and birth—they saw their brother's birth with their own eyes—but they were still totally astounded by what we told them. We were explaining puberty and the menstrual cycle (involving "the egg that isn't fertilized"), and then my husband explained that sex is when a man puts his penis in a woman's vagina and moves it back and forth until sperm shoots out and sometimes a sperm meets the egg and makes a baby. Abram asked a few practical questions, like "How many squirts?" But Moses looked completely horrified.

"It feels good," I told Moses.

"How do *you* know?" asked Abram.

My husband and I looked at each other, confused. We'd just explained to them that this is how babies are made. And there we were sitting with our two sons at dinner, our third son asleep in the other room.

"Because we've done it," Josh said.

"You *did* that? You *did*? I *never* saw you do that!" said Abram in disbelief.

Now the baby is single-mindedly trying to console himself

at my breast. I'll give him a nice long bath in the big tub with me—he always loves that.

* *

Reading *Gregor the Overlander* to the big boys.

* *

When he was nine months old, my son Moses stopped nursing. At six months he started crawling, and after that it was hard for him to nurse. Every time I got him settled, he'd nurse for a minute, then pull away. He preferred the bottle, which he could drink while looking around. I tried nursing him in a quiet room, but no room seemed quiet enough. There was always something he wanted to see or do. We struggled for a few weeks until nursing was no longer a sweet, intimate time but a battle of wills. My dogged attempts to make him nurse—jamming my breast in his mouth, coaxing him gently and then not so gently to turn towards me—started to feel almost abusive. Finally the pediatrician asked, "Who are you doing this for—you or him? He doesn't seem to want it." So I stopped. Within a month I was pregnant with Abram.

I thought Abram would nurse forever. He refused a bottle for his first eight months, but then at nine months he refused the breast, just as Moses had done. He was starting daycare, so I decided not to fight it, and in a few days' time he was weaned.

Tonight I feel a shard of doubt about my determination to nurse Judah for at least a year. Here I am, living in a place and among people who support breastfeeding. My supply is good, my health is strong, my schedule is flexible. I don't intend to send this baby to daycare until he is at least fifteen months old. But, even in these circumstances, nursing isn't always easy, and it's not always what I want to be doing. I'm tied to the baby. My sex drive is muted. My hair is falling out. My right shoulder hurts every time I raise my arm above my waist. I still leak through my bras and shirts. I have to be careful about what I eat and drink. I often feel like the illustration above the caption "He was sucking the life out of her."

As a mother, I'm not free. Judah depends on me, and my body, in many ways, still belongs to him. Even if I weren't nursing, I would be tied to him, but nursing makes our connection inescapable. Nursing makes the relationship I have with my baby concrete. Maybe I need that. Maybe I need the quiet room as much as he does.

* *

At the pediatrician's office, where the baby is getting the pneumococcal vaccination.

* *

At the Upper Breast Side store, getting fitted for nursing bras.

* *

Having lunch with my friend Erin and baby James.

* *

At my mother's appointment with a cardiologist.

*   *

Having dinner with the three boys.

*   *

I've nursed several times today without writing. I haven't
wanted to write or wanted to nurse, but I've had to nurse. The
pain in my shoulder has gotten worse. Even though it's October,
it's 85 degrees and humid. The baby hasn't pooped for over a
week and is cranky. I had hoped this project would inspire me
or at least yield interesting material. I imagined dreamily poetic
discourse written in periodic fragments, which would elucidate
the process of nursing in some visceral way. All I've managed
with this nursing journal is a litany of banalities, and the process
feels like a burden. I have to nurse when I'm not really in the
mood and now I have to write about it, too. But what should I
have written about while nursing? Politics? Literary criticism?

A memory just came back to me: When I was four months
post partum with Abram, I went to see a psychiatrist. I had two
children under two, had just dropped out of a graduate program
I liked, was waiting to find out if my book would be accepted
for publication, and Bush had just "won" the election recount.
It was a dark time. I'd heard that this psychiatrist specialized in
postpartum depression and knew which antidepressants one
could safely take while nursing. I talked and cried, and she listened. Finally, she wrote me a prescription and recommended
that at least once a day I nurse without doing anything else.
No reading, talking on the phone, or watching TV. "Just look
at the baby," she said. I thought her suggestion was condescending and belittling. Didn't she understand I felt trapped? I

felt overwhelmed by my children and the responsibilities of caring for them. Only while nursing did I have time to read or watch TV or talk on the phone. I craved these things, needed them. I didn't take her advice, and I didn't take the medication she prescribed. In time, things improved.

Four months after Judah's birth, life is very full. Sometimes I feel harassed and annoyed, but I'm not depressed. I am indescribably grateful for my three healthy boys and for the privilege of being able to raise them with my husband. The psychiatrist's advice comes back to me tonight, almost seven years later, and I'm finally ready to hear it. I often do other things while nursing. In fact, it would be easier for me to write a list of things that I *haven't* done while nursing, but this obsession with multi-tasking is not good for me. The past three days of writing while nursing have unbalanced me. Part of the joy of having an infant is the permission to enter—the necessity of entering—the nonverbal, preintellectual, animal realm. Nursing is a portal to the mind's quiet room, to Babyland, where the entertainment is the sunlight moving across the wall, and the only things on the schedule are eating and sleeping. Only the baby has nowhere to go. I'll put down my pen, watch him suck, and let him take me there.

⁎

Rachel Zucker is the author of three books of poetry (*The Bad Wife Handbook*, *The Last Clear Narrative*, and *Eating in the Underworld*), coeditor of *Women Poets on Mentorship: Efforts and Affections*, and coauthor of *Home/Birth*. Zucker has taught poetry and writing at several universities and is a certified labor doula. She lives in New York City with her husband and three sons.

STEP ONE, TRY IT; STEP TWO, WHATEVER WORKS

Paula Spencer

"Want me to take him to the nursery so you can get some sleep?"

I glance from the postpartum nurse to the still-unreal bundle in my arms. Henry. My son. There's a nursery here? I'd picked this hospital for my delivery partly for its policy of having newborns "room in" with their mothers. Rooming-in was one of those items on the get-ready-for-baby checklists I'd lived by that sounded as critical as it was amorphous and alien, like burp cloths or car-seat installation. It had something to do with bonding.

Back when I was researching state-of-the-art birthing centers, though, I hadn't counted on spending thirty-nine straight hours awake—a day at work, an evening rabidly cleaning out the linen closet for the first time ever, then a long night and a morning in labor, followed by a packed day, counting and recounting fingers and toes while making giddy phone calls. Adrenaline had powered me through that last part. Then it abruptly left the building an hour ago, along with my exhausted husband.

Take him to the nursery? Hey, you're the expert. All I know about babies is what I read in books.

"Sure," I say.

There is no painful, ripping Velcro sound as my baby separates from my arms. There is only quiet, and the relief of imminent sleep. I'm too tired to care that barely twelve hours into motherhood I've already veered perilously off course.

Technically I'd messed up my candidacy for Mother Supreme even before the umbilical cord quit pulsing. Left to his own devices, a fresh-from-the-womb newborn will inch up his mother's body to find her breast and latch on, following an instinct as potent as any wolf pup's in the wild. Or so said my dog-eared copy of *The Amazing Newborn*. For nine months I'd pored over its black-and-white photos like a pioneer agog over pamphlets about the Promised Land to the west. I couldn't wait to see this marsupial creep for myself. I'd see if my baby turned to his daddy's voice, supposedly as familiar as my own from the womb, as the book said. I would make an O with my mouth and watch my baby imitate it while just minutes old.

In the silent pages of the book, however, there was no jubilant kissing and telephoning going on. There was no hysterical baby boy howling through his cleanup and weigh-in. My fellow was amazing, all right, just not in a social-science kind of way.

After four hours of getting used to him and four thousand photos, the hospital's lactation consultant came by to ask if he'd nursed yet. Ah, feed him! We'd been too busy counting fingers and toes as he slept and saying, "Ohmygodwehaveababy!" Feeding him hadn't crossed my mind. She planted his tiny head next to a breast twice its circumference (mine, speaking of amazing) and gave us a quick lesson in latching on. The duet came naturally. Well, aside from those few days until my tender nipples adjusted to this new kind of use, when I bit a washcloth every time he hungrily clamped down.

For the record, that first night in the nursery Henry didn't appear to miss me, either. The nurses did not feed him a bottle of sugar-water, as the pro-rooming-in tracts had warned they might. At least, nobody told me he got sugar-water, and I do have fuzzy memories of being awakened to nurse once or twice. But the nurses could have fed him coconut milk for all I cared that night, so long as they did him no harm. The enormity of bringing someone into a room through my body, not the door, made the tangential details shrink to a shrug. Forgetting to bring that favorite T-shirt to labor in? My hospital gown worked fine. My fancy for squatting to push the baby out during delivery? It had evaporated when I needed three people just to hold up my shaky legs while I lay on my back. Then I had an episiotomy *and* a huge tear; so much for perineal massage.

Rooming-in, like putting the baby to the breast during the supposedly critical first hour of life, was just another abandoned ideal that suddenly didn't seem remotely important. I had sleep. The baby was still alive. So far, so good.

Once we are home, a precious pot of New Zealand lanolin becomes my new best friend. I stock up on shirts with hidden openings and spend contented hours in my glider rocker, a water bottle at my side. I learn to nurse confidently in public— in cars, on planes, on trains (and possibly while reciting Dr. Seuss aloud in the rain). I can even suckle while simultaneously typing and talking on the phone, a breastfeeding hold described in no guide I've devoured.

When Henry is four weeks old, he outgrows the heirloom cradle next to our bed and I relocate him to a crib in his own room, down the hall. A few weeks later he's sleeping through the night (or from 10:00 P.M. to 4:00 or 5:00 A.M., which by this point is nirvana, not to mention a reasonable facsimile of "all night"). Then, at three and a half months, my champion sleeper begins backsliding. Goodbye, blissful six hours of sleep in a row. My mom tells me to mix a little cereal with formula and feed it before bedtime. I ask my pediatrician what he thinks. My pediatrician tells me to mix a little cereal with formula and feed it before bedtime. He's been a pediatrician for as long as my mom has raised five kids. It works.

I also leave the occasional bottle of half-and-half (half formula, half me) or a can of ready-to-pour Similac for babysitters or his daycare "teachers." I try to express a few extra ounces for this before or after work, though only when I have both time and inclination. Fortunately the baby is in a corporate child-care center near my office, so I don't have to miss many feedings. I slip out at mealtimes and get discreet phone calls to hurry if I'm delayed. If I had to pump several times a day (or more ambitiously, FedEx milk back home from business trips, as colleagues do), I'm sure I wouldn't have bothered pumping at all, no matter how clean and private the pumping room or how understanding my boss. Without snuggling in the equation, making milk hardly seems worth the bother, especially since most of those protective antibodies entered his system in the earliest weeks of the business. Despite my slightly erratic production schedule, my milk supply never shrivels to the point of sudden infant starvation.

Naturally, I consider myself a "breastfeeding mother." A successful one at that. I nurse Henry for six months, long past the national average.

Too bad that virtually every preceding sentence brands me a loser at the job, according to prevailing winds of advice and expectation that have whipped up the definition of *breastfeeding mother* to intimidating proportions. Sure, sure, "breast is best." But in just the fifteen years since I whipped out my first colostrum-rich nipple, breastfeeding advocates have raised the bar so high on what counts as the right way to feed a baby, it's a wonder anybody dares to start.

Especially after she faces the much-hyped recommendation that breastfeeding ought to continue for a marathon twelve months. A full year of breastfeeding is a tall order when the typical maternity leave lasts six weeks. Emphasizing the endpoint (*You really ought to do this for twelve months*) makes the whole prospect a lot less inviting than lowering the bar to *Give it a try because your breasts will fill with milk anyway and it's really good for your baby even if you do it for just a day or two*. Anybody might be game to give it a day. Making a commitment for a full year when you can't even think straight is like sending yourself an invitation to feeling like Failure Mom should you slack off at any point along the way, for whatever reason.

What's more, there's little talk of combining breast and formula (or, heaven forbid, milk and solid food) to keep it going. Today moms are routinely advised to lay off the Gerber for six months. And formula may as well be devil juice.

Another apparent mistake I made: all those working lunches and dinners using my patented multi-tasking breast-feeding hold. The new thinking is to use feeding times as an opportunity to stimulate your baby's brain cells by making eye contact and chatting, not to preserve your own by getting caught up on the news. *Your* needs? *Your* sleep? How dare you be so selfish!

Woe, too, to the hapless new mom whose circle of peers includes someone a little too intoxicated with sharing news of the dangers of phthalates in plastic bottles or the politics of co-sleeping, after spending a few too many hours plugged into the more paranoid corners of the momosphere. Childbirth-class re-unions that should be spent comparing stretch marks or devel-opmental milestones—or, better yet, exchanging tips on how to avoid getting sucked into work before your leave is up—de-scend into harangues or debates. No, girlfriend, I don't want to donate leftovers to the local human milk bank.

Back when I became a nursing mother, "attachment par-enting" was still just the name of a chapter Dr. William Sears threw into one of his books, not a lifestyle with rules (and busy-bodies) of its own. Nobody was organizing "lactivists" into suckle-ins every time an intimidated mother collided with an ill-informed shopkeeper over her right to feed her baby wher-ever she chose. I've fed my kids while wedged between two businessmen on a United Airlines flight, in Sunday school, and even during business meetings. I was discreet and nobody ever gaped, much less showed me to the door, though if they had I'd have rolled my eyes and said, "Grow up." Although a decade ago there were the occasional headline-making arrests over public nursing, the issue hadn't yet been trumped up into a civil-rights campaign.

It's a shame, really. Instead of being a natural extension of pregnancy and childbirth, something you just *do* right away to pass on all those protective antibodies (and save a little cash at a time when it's flying out of your wallet as if it had been sprin-kled with pixie dust back there in the delivery room), breast-feeding has been turned into a statement. A chore. Another series of tests on the way to "good" motherhood.

I breastfed because I was convinced it was a smart start. I kept at it because it was much more pleasurable than I'd imag-ined (not that one can accurately imagine much about breast-feeding before actually doing it). I made it work for me. And then when my baby grew teeth and I grew tired of being tethered to the baby or the pump, I quit.

The message to new moms and mothers-to-be should be, Take breastfeeding one day at a time. Try it in the hospital—you're just lying there anyway. And people there are glad to show you how. Stick it out during maternity leave to pass all those health benefits to your baby, and to yourself. Plus, it's free, and it's easier to stuff a ready nipple into a hungry mouth than to prep a bottle every hour while suffering extreme sleep deprivation.

And then—see how it goes. Maybe it will be easier, and more enjoyable, than you thought, the way it was for me. Maybe you'll move on in a few weeks or months. Maybe you'll stick with this feeding option right through toddlerhood. Whatever follows, everybody will be okay.

That's the real definition of success: everybody coming out okay.

Henry is not a week old when I'm home explaining for the twentieth time to my husband, George, that no, breastfeeding does not feel erotic. (Has he never noticed I manage nicely through foreplay without gritting my teeth into a Turkish towel?) The doorbell rings. Again. It's not that I don't appreciate the chance to show off our son. (*Our son!*) But I'm jangly from new-mom fatigue, insecurity, and the soreness of ten thousand stitches somewhere I can't quite place on my shell-shocked lower body. Visits wear me out. Blessedly, most friends and neighbors coo at Henry, bestow a bib or a Onesie (or, even better, a ready-to-eat lasagne), and split.

Barbara brings beer.

"Here's a welcome-home present just for you." She sets down a wrapped six-pack of Michelob. "My pediatrician's wife brought me some after Anna was born. She said it's good for the let-down reflex."

My milk comes in—and goes out—just fine. But the rest of me could use a little unwinding. If a pediatrician's wife said so, it must be okay, right? I gladly down half a bottle. I do not "pump and dump the milk that is most affected by the drink," as a government website admonishes. Henry does not develop fetal alcohol syndrome. And I really do feel much more relaxed.

In fact, the boy, now a teenager, has gone on to perfect health, with nary a food allergy or ounce of excess fat. He makes the A-B honor roll and once got the Presidential Physical Fitness Award. He towers over me and looks his dad in the eye. At eight, he made me a card: "To the best Mommy I ever had." We're bonded very nicely, thanks.

Same for his three younger sisters—despite the fact that I stuck each of them in a room down the hall at night and weaned them to fake milk before they were five months old. I never even warmed up the bottles. Then again, I never preheated their baby food—or their diaper wipes—either.

I did, however, chill the Michelob. It was good.

☀

Paula Spencer is the author of Momfidence: An Oreo Never Killed Anybody and Other Secrets of Happier Parenting, the "Momfidence" columnist for Woman's Day magazine, and a longtime contributing editor of Parenting and Babytalk. She lives with her husband and their four children in Chapel Hill, North Carolina.

MOTHERHOOD MADE
A LIAR OUT OF ME

Daryn Eller

"Is she weaned?"

It was a casual question asked by a woman whose daughter was playing next to my thirteen-month-old in the sand. "Yes," I said, giving a casual—and deceitful—reply.

Technically, it was only a little lie: Aidan wasn't really weaned because I had never breastfed her a day in her young life. But it felt monumental to me. With that one little lie I had not only made myself seem like someone I had always hoped to be—a nurturing, lactating mom—but I had also successfully stifled my usual urge to talk a blue streak on the subject.

For too long I'd been telling the truth, and I mean the *whole* truth, by which I mean the entire story about why I hadn't breastfed Aidan. Another mother on the playground would ask a simple question and I'd launch into my life story. It was a compulsion; I couldn't stop myself, even though, inevitably, at story's end I'd be asking myself, "Why did I just reveal very personal information to a complete stranger?" It wasn't information that I was ashamed of—quite the contrary—but since I'm normally fairly reticent, my openness would ultimately make me uncomfortable. Afterwards, pushing my daughter in her stroller on the way home, I'd feel like I'd just gone to a party, taken my clothes off, and jumped into the pool.

The main reason I didn't breastfeed Aidan is that she's adopted. Most people don't know that you can breastfeed an adopted baby, so anytime anyone asked me about nursing I could have just said, "My daughter's adopted," and left it at that. But I didn't. Because I knew that it's possible to breastfeed an adopted baby, I always felt as if further explanation was needed. Maybe I'd read too much propaganda about how absolutely important nursing is for a child's health and for mother-baby bonding, but I couldn't help worrying that others would judge me for not going the extra mile.

I know, it sounds paranoid, but of course this wasn't really about what other people thought of me. It was about what I thought of me. Even though I believed that my reasons for not breastfeeding were legitimate, I still felt guilty about it. And I also felt sort of left out. No matter how much I love my daughter—and believe me, my love for her is deep and indelible—as a mother I will always feel as though I'm a little different from the other members of the club.

It's a club I had really, really wanted to belong to, and once I had the credentials—that is, a baby in tow—I made a concerted effort to join. I took Aidan to the park almost every day, even when she was tiny, just so she could look at the bigger kids and so I, I hoped, could connect with other mothers. We went to a weekly music "class," attended library story hours, and signed up for gym 'n' swim at the Y. And it worked. Each step of the way, I met women with infants the same age as mine, and I loved it. With my badges earned for sleepless nights, spit-up-stained clothes, and hours spent walking a fussing baby around the house, I finally felt like a full-fledged member of the moms' club.

Except when I didn't. Those were the times when I'd be hanging out with a group and the conversation would turn to pregnancy or breastfeeding. I couldn't do much about the fact that my daughter hadn't gestated inside my own uterus, but breastfeeding was different; that had actually been within my control, and I'd opted out. So whenever a klatch of moms started talking about breast pumps and nursing bras (and believe me, during the first year they always do), I would either quietly scoot Aidan over to the swings, decide it was a good time to take pity on the lone dad in the park (he and I had something in common, after all), or tell my story. "Oh, I'm not breastfeeding," I would say, and open the faucet.

I had no time to consider breastfeeding, I'd tell them, because I'd left the house one morning not expecting anything of consequence to happen and came home the next day with a baby. On the day of Aidan's birth, I had actually flown to a spa in Tucson to do a magazine piece on meditation (something I actually hate), but before I could unpack my bag or utter a single *om*, my husband, Andy, called to tell me he'd heard from our adoption attorney. Aidan's birth mother was in labor and on her way to the hospital and had called him to say she needed a family for her baby. Though she knew she wanted to give up her child, she never contacted anyone to arrange an adoption until she was literally en route to the delivery room. After our lawyer read profiles of all his clients to her over the phone, she chose us. My husband drove the forty-five minutes to the hospital, I got on the next plane out of Tucson, and we spent the night in a room on the maternity ward, our daughter asleep on my chest.

Because we went from people hoping to adopt a baby, but with no prospects in sight, to parents of a newborn in the space of a couple of hours, we didn't have a minute to prepare for getting a bassinet, let alone for breastfeeding. I didn't know much about how you go about breastfeeding an adopted baby; I had heard you could only a few months before from my friend Toni, another adoptive mother. When Toni and her husband, Rich, were at the hospital waiting to take home their adopted daughter, a woman they'd never seen before approached them and asked Toni, "You're going to breastfeed her, aren't you?" Toni's head was already spinning—she had a newborn daughter!—and the woman was bullying and aggressive. Toni and Rich couldn't get away from her fast enough.

When Toni told me about what happened, I was just as incredulous as she was. How rude! I thought. Still, the possibility that you could breastfeed an adopted baby hovered on the edges of my mind. It was an interesting idea, but I let it drop. I wasn't ready to think about it or, for that matter, anything else that had to do with taking care of an infant.

If you're preparing to adopt, it probably makes good sense to prepare for life with a child. Yet I couldn't help feeling that it would be pathetic to sit there with an empty crib, gazing up into the stars and wishing for my dreams to come true. I'm just not the type. So while I was optimistic I also remained cautious; I just didn't want to get my hopes up too high. I remember one couple in our adoption prep class, two lovely men, telling us that their dining room table was covered with baby gifts just waiting for their future bundle of joy—even though, at the time, they had already been turned down by a few birth mothers. I wondered how they felt looking at those gifts each time a potential adoption fell through.

We had one disappointment of our own that made me approach the whole endeavor with caution. After an impromptu phone conversation with a birth mother who was just days away from giving birth, we hopped in the car and traveled across the state to meet her (she was a lawyer, Jewish like us—the presumably intelligent and genetically companionable birth mother we could only have dreamed of). Andy and I had dinner with her and her ten-year-old daughter, and we really hit it off. It seemed a fait accompli. The next morning, after a reassuring phone conversation, we headed home, contemplating girls' names as we drove down Highway 5, only to get a call from our attorney telling us the birth mother had changed her mind and decided to go with the family to whom she'd originally promised the baby. Imagine if we'd come home to an empty baby's room. Instead, we never bought so much as a diaper or a baby book, and our guest room remained just that, a guest room.

Once we had an actual live baby on our hands, breastfeeding was the last thing on my mind. I had to figure out all of the rest of the stuff, including who was going to care for her while I worked part time. So I didn't think about breastfeeding until I started venturing out and talking to other moms. Everyone seemed to be talking about breastfeeding, and there was pro-nursing propaganda everywhere. Before we even left the hospital we had to endure a video presentation for new parents, 75 percent of which dealt with nursing (we were relieved when they finally got to the swaddling and diapering part). And the messages weren't just for mothers who gave birth: Even the American Academy of Pediatrics had revised its position on breastfeeding to include a recommendation that physicians help adoptive parents learn how to breastfeed their babies. (This, by the way, entails pumping for several weeks and possibly taking a drug to help promote milk production. And most times this won't produce enough of a supply to avoid supplementation with formula.) One day when I was sitting on a bench giving Aidan a bottle at an open-air mall, a ragged homeless man admonished me for not breastfeeding (I'm not making this up). Reflexively, I started to explain, only to catch myself when I realized the ridiculousness of it all.

So, was formula feeding so bad? Um, no, though I still worried. During the first two years of her life, Aidan didn't seem to get sick more than any other kid I knew, but whenever she had an ear infection—two, maybe three times—I would feel a little tug at my heart: Was it because I didn't breastfeed? Bonding was different; it was happening, breast or no breast, and we shared and still share, now that she is edging towards age four, a physical closeness. This has given me a little more understanding of why many women love breastfeeding. The weight of your child against you is like no other form of touch that I know. It's why, despite her age and size (and despite advice to the contrary), I often carry Aidan the whole quarter mile home from preschool. (At least it's all downhill. I draw the line at carrying her *to* school.)

Along with things like not having to sit in your car and pump, as one friend told me she used to do because there was no privacy in her office, there are advantages to not breastfeeding, even for the child. Aidan has always been as attached to Andy as she is to me. She rarely has wanted just Mommy, and I think this has something to do with the fact that Andy fed her almost as often as I did. When you're not nursing, your significant other has no excuse for not doing equal time. Andy couldn't hear Aidan cry in the night, turn over, and legitimately leave the feeding to me. He had to do his part, and he did.

One of the ironic facts of my nonbreastfeeding life is that the mother of Aidan's best friend, Claudia, who has become one of my own closest friends, breastfed her daughter until she was well past the age of three. I love Leticia for many reasons, but mostly because she is an open book. Consequently, she was constantly talking to me about her struggles with weaning Claudia. She wanted to, she said, but she always had an excuse as to why she hadn't. Sometimes I felt like channeling Nancy Reagan and yelling, "Just say no!" But as a nonnurser I didn't really have a leg to stand on. I could tell, though, that despite her protests to the contrary, she really didn't want to stop breastfeeding. She worked all day, and nursing Claudia helped assuage some of the guilt of being away.

All this advanced-age breastfeeding was not lost on Aidan, who began to take notice that Claudia was getting something she wasn't. She started asking me for *teta*, Spanish for "breast" (Leticia is Cuban), then lifting my shirt and sucking on my stomach (clearly she didn't know what *teta* really was). I loved this, but, as I was not able to deliver, it also embarrassed me a little.

After a while, as our kids got older, all the talk about breastfeeding seemed to die down. I didn't have to lie anymore, save for the infrequent conversation with a pregnant or brand-new mother, when I would just nod my head as if to say, "Oh, yeah, been there, done that." Then, three of the moms in our play group had second babies, and talk once again turned to breast pumps and nursing bras. But, funnily enough, it wasn't long before these conversations turned to weaning—they were all determined to do a shorter stint breastfeeding this time around.

Even Leticia. Anticipating her return to work, she turned to me one day, her new son just one month old, and said, "I need to talk to you about formula."

✳

Daryn Eller is a freelance writer whose work has appeared in *Parents*, *Parenting*, *O: The Oprah Magazine*, *Prevention*, and *Health* magazines. She is the coauthor of *Rooms to Grow In: Little Folk Art's Great Rooms for Babies, Kids, and Teens* (Clarkson Potter, 2001). She lives in Venice, California.

SWL(ACTATING)F SEEKING SEX WITH NO STRINGS ATTACHED

Rachel Sarah

On Thanksgiving Day my boyfriend walked out the door. Our daughter was seven months old, and I'll never know for sure what put him over the edge. He was bipolar. He drank. He was fragile. He didn't leave a forwarding address.

This was a time when I believed that love would overcome anything. Well, it certainly overcame me. The very first thing I did, even before crying, was to sit down on the living room rug and nurse my daughter, Mae. Nursing was my landing pad. It was the place where my milk could turn my anger into white, warm calmness. Nursing had the same soothing effect on my baby, no matter how hungry, agitated, red-faced, and cranky she was at the start. Nothing beat nursing.

No matter how alone I felt, those times that Mae lay on my chest, her tiny hands kneading my breasts, milk flowing from me, I knew that I could do this alone. Not only did nursing nourish Mae, it nourished me. But it wasn't long after her father split town—as Mae's first birthday approached without a sign from him, I knew he wasn't coming back—that friends started to ask me, "When are you going to get back out there?"

As in *date?* They had to be kidding. Not only was I a twenty-nine-year-old single mom with dishes in the sink and baby clothes with stains I'd never actually scrub out, but I breastfed "on demand." How in the world could I even think about hooking up with some hot man when my cha-chas were making milk?

*   *

"But look at you!" my girlfriends (who were all married) said to me. "You're attractive, and you're young."

Maybe they were right. About getting back out there, anyway. As the months passed, I started to notice men: our building manager—who gave Mae stuffed animals and called her "Little Guacamole"—and the UPS man, who rolled his packages past me.

Still, noticing men in the hallway was *not* the same as dating them. I'm grateful that back then I did not sit down at my computer and type *lactating and dating* into Google. If I had, I *never* would have gone on a date. Because recently, while writing this essay, I turned to my computer to do some research, in hopes of finding a thoughtful example of what it means to balance these two acts. I hoped to come across a first-person essay in *Redbook* about a mother's deep feelings, something to inspire me as I worked.

One of the first things that came up, however, was a site called MilkMyTits.com. Men were looking for "mature women willing to breastfeed me."

Gross. I kept scrolling through the sites that Google brought up; there *had* to be something. But they were all the same: white men in their forties in search of sweet breast milk.

My breasts had always been one of the most sensual parts of me. Before motherhood, when a man put his lips around my nipple, it made my body rain—not a light sprinkle, either. If I slept with a man as a nursing mom, my breasts would rain on him. Perhaps, after undressing, I could open my closet, pull out an umbrella, and hand it to him: "You might need this . . ."

I couldn't remember if I'd slept with Mae's father in the weeks before he'd left for good. If I had, I didn't remember the details. He was shut down and hung-over; I was absorbed with my baby. I lived in the world of womanhood for years, and now I was a mother. But who says that you can't live in both worlds? Some mothers I knew wore bras to bed because they didn't want to leak on the mattress—or their husbands. That's how they divided their realms. But I wanted to be a woman who lived in both worlds; I wanted to be the kind of woman who didn't care if she spurted.

One of my best friends in New York City told me that she wanted to set me up on a blind date. Ironically, she was the same friend who, in 2002, was thrown out of the public library in Manhattan for breastfeeding her daughter. She'd been nursing in an empty reading room, when a female security guard screamed at her to "take that outside." The guard didn't know that my friend, Susan Light, was a lawyer who took it straight to the media, after which the library expressed "deep regret" over the incident and immediately sent a memo to remind staff of the right of women to breastfeed.

"I want to date, but I can't," I told my friend.

"Why not?"

"I'm nursing."

"So?" she said.

"What would I wear?" I huffed. "A nursing bra?"

She laughed.

"No, really," I said. "I'd have to bring my pump along, for after my drink."

Little did my mother-friend know that the blind date she wanted to set me up with might have had a breastfeeding fetish. She told me that he was a lawyer, too, "a cute one." After chatting on the phone with the lawyer his call woke me as I fell asleep while nursing Mae in the bed we share—I decided to go for it. I've always considered myself to be open-minded about anything intimate. Maybe I was rebelling against my Catholic mother, but I certainly was not a prude. I decided that I'd keep the date short and sweet—and I'd nurse before leaving so (I hoped) I wouldn't leak.

The following Friday, after enlisting another girlfriend to baby-sit, I dashed out the door to meet the lawyer at a bar. When I got inside, he waved. I didn't see the cuteness—he had a receding hairline—but maybe I was too nervous.

Still, he did the right thing: He asked if I had a photo of Mae, and when I pulled one from my wallet, he used the word *adorable*.

"She is," I said. "I'm late because I was nursing her before bed—"

"You were nursing her?"

That's when I noticed the sparkle in his eyes. Maybe I'd misread? But no.

"A woman who's lactating!" he said, way too loudly. "What a turn-on!"

I waited for the punch line, but he was not joking. I've always had this untactful knack for blurting out details that shock people—I do it without thinking. Why did I tell him that I was breastfeeding? Nursing was such an essential part of who I was, it was like telling someone, "The sitter was running late, I'm sorry—"

It's always *after* the fact when I realize I should be wearing a soft muzzle. The lawyer's enthusiasm was a sure giveaway that I'd said too much. I didn't know if I should crawl under the table or give him a high-five. Was I flattered or freaked out? Or a little of both?

But the truth was, if any possible romantic date of mine was squeamish about the fact that I was breastfeeding, I did need to know this up front. I mean, if I hadn't said anything, and then all of a sudden he looked down and noticed the wet spots on my blouse, that would have been interesting.

And that's exactly what happened.

If you've ever breastfed, you know that just thinking about nursing can, well, have certain consequences. My breasts were flooding with milk. I had no control over it, and when I looked down, there was a damp spot on my chest.

Maybe it was all in the name of discovery, but perhaps more important, I liked the fact that this man acknowledged who I was: a woman *as well as* a nursing mother. He could have overlooked that wet spot on my blouse. He could have glanced at his watch, embarrassed, and said, "I'd better get home."

At the time I wasn't interested in having him—or anyone, for that matter—as a companion. I was an unseasoned single mom who was trying to get over her ex. I was still trying to get a handle on raising my daughter solo. I wasn't ready for a relationship. But I *did* crave sex. And I was curious. I wanted to know what it felt like to have a man drink my milk.

Afterwards, when I told a couple of friends what had happened, they scrunched their noses up. "You let him do *what?*"

Much to the dismay of my girlfriend who was babysitting,

I brought him home. As my daughter slept in the other room, I let him unbutton my blouse and run his mouth across the edge of my bra. I let him touch me. When I started to leak, he was ecstatic. He told me that he'd never tasted anything so sweet in his life. (Yes, I wondered if, maybe, his mother had never breastfed him.) But this is what mattered most: He wanted me as I was, and I didn't have to hide any of it.

✳

Rachel Sarah's book *Single Mom Seeking: Playdates, Blind Dates and Other Dispatches from the Dating World* was published in 2007. Rachel is the single-mom columnist for LifetimeTV.com, and she has written for *Family Circle*, *Pregnancy*, *Parenting*, *Literary Mama*, BabyCenter.com, and *American Baby*.

TIT FOR TAT

Leslie Crawford

Before we were mothers together, Kirstin and I were little more than casual friends. She was a friend of a friend, but sharing a closer bond never seemed possible. She resided in a different stratosphere. Kirstin was authentically blond, a six-figure accountant with strapping, Swedish good looks. She ran five miles a day, wrote and published a novel in her spare time, had an adorable son, and, I was sure, wore lacy underwear that always matched. In comparison, I felt thoroughly unremarkable.

But when we both learned we were pregnant, she with her second, I with my first, and due within days of each other in September, our relationship instantly changed. What with my freckled Irish face, small and unspectacular frame, and low-paying job as an editor, I knew I could never match her when it came to cheekbones or ambition or expensive shoes. But now we shared something deeply intimate, something that finally put me on solid footing: motherhood.

Since we lived within blocks of one another, Kirstin suggested we take walks together at 6:00 A.M.: two pregnant women keeping each other company and keeping fit. I was thankful for her initiative and accepted, figuring because of our respective girths I'd be able to keep up with her otherwise manic marathon pace. So we began our morning ritual. Our walks marked the beginning of a blossoming and lasting friendship, one that grew at once stronger and more competitive (competitive on my side, anyway) because of motherhood. Maybe Kirstin's perfection brought out my competitive streak, but I think I can share some of the blame with society at large: Once a woman is with child, her worth is determined by how good a mother she is. Prove you're not just good, but the best—the Mother of all mothers—and, even if you were never cheerleader or prom queen, you've won the grand prize.

So began my stealth mission to prove myself when my son was not even the size of a tangerine. When Kirstin began preparing her daughter's nursery and pulled out the crib she'd used for her son, I explained with all the inflated piousness of a zealot that our child would sleep with my husband and me rather than be confined to a mini-prison. Instead of stuffing him in a stroller as Kirstin did her older son, I would "wear" my baby at all times, close to my warm, beating heart. I announced I would nurse my baby as long as he wanted, whenever he wanted. Kirstin, I noted scornfully, had breastfed her son for only a year, if that. My hooters may not have been nearly as lovely as hers, but on the breastfeeding front, I'd be the winner. If Kirstin was annoyed by my self-righteous rants, she never showed it. Geez, not only was this woman beautiful, she was gracious and kind, too.

This was years ago, when baby slings and family beds were more marginal than mainstream, before Sears replaced Spock as the guru for a new generation of militant moms. Back then, I was a mother-to-be on the sanctimonious fringe, having read every possible book on nouveau parenting, including one about women from an Amazonian tribe who raised blissed-out children because they carried their babies every moment during their infant's first year.

"Oh, please," my husband, Steve, said when I parroted the same propaganda to him that I did to Kirstin. "They carry their babies so they don't fall off cliffs or get eaten by snakes." I pooh-poohed the skepticism and, once Sam was born, carried him every second of the day when I wasn't at work. Naturally, Sam wore cloth diapers, while Kirstin's baby wore those toxic, Elmo-stamped paper ones. Bad mom. Good mom.

I might even brag that as Sam grew into a plump, healthy baby, fed on nothing but my prodigious milk, which he seemed to drink nonstop, I more than excelled at nursing. What a superstar breastfeeder I was, an achievement I could finally be proud of! I have such a short list of things that make me exceptional. I am great at jumping rope, having learned from a pro boxer actually named Rocky. I'm a terrifically fast typist. I'm an expert lap swimmer. There is a pattern here. I'm accomplished at repetitive skills that can be hard to master. After I suffer the pain and the calluses, whether on my heels, fingers, or nipples, I'm hard to beat.

That is, until the terrible day that I discovered Kirstin had out-pumped me. She and I had decided to share her babysitter. After settling Sam in the living room with her daughter, Tessa, and the sitter, I went to deposit my "liquid gold" in the freezer. This is the contradictory part of being a modern mother: By claiming your independence, working or doing things away from your baby, you transform yourself into an industrial farm sow/cow. And there's nothing more bovine than hooking yourself up to a sterile machine to stockpile milk for your baby while you're away.

How can I properly convey my horror that Monday morning as I stood, frozen in place by the insult of it all, staring into Kirstin's freezer. There, lined up like so much plastic-encased artillery prepared for an attack, were rows upon rows of her frozen breast milk. Each neat white bullet had been dutifully dated in indelible black pen and was filled precisely to the same line. My God! Where were the pints of Ben & Jerry's, the staple of a nursing mother's diet? Absent, too, were the frozen pizzas, the half-empty bags of peas, the freezer-burned lasagne leftovers. All else that remained in that Siberian snow-white desert of milk, and more milk, was a tray of ice cubes.

Life is so unfair.

Up to this moment I had claimed my unspoken victory as Mother Superior over my otherwise far superior friend. Now she had beaten me in the battle of the breast milk, an arena in which I thought I'd claimed an unquestioned victory. As I continued staring at the brutal evidence of her milky prowess, clutching my five bags that were the sum total of my pumped milk and pondering where to insert my paltry offering in her vast lactation warehouse, I wondered: Who is this wonder woman, this Valkyrie of the milk barn?

"This is war," I told Steve that night, to the *whir-whir* of my black Medela pump. I went on a milking binge, pumping so much from my overworked breasts that I transformed into a one-woman milk farm. At home at night, I'd stay awake after Sam's feedings to pump. At work, during coffee breaks and lunchtime and in between, I stole away to one of the two single bathrooms in our trendy, industrial-chic loft offices, the obscene moaning of my black Medela making me feel somehow furtive, like a pervert doing something unseemly behind locked doors. Where once I was a model workaholic, I'd become a pumpaholic, filling up one glorious bag after another.

How triumphant I felt on the days I'd stride confidently into Kirstin's house to drop off Sam, continuing into the kitchen to claim my expanding territory in her freezer. I was sure to always neatly label my many milk bags, proudly leaving my mark, "LC," with a date underneath. (As our combined collection amassed, I'd worry that the sitter, Monika, who was given to fits of passive-aggressive snippiness, might give Sam Kirstin's milk, just to spite me, like a bitter chef who spits in the soup.)

Perhaps because of my newfound confidence, I let down my guard and was able to enjoy Kirstin more. I grew to see beyond her looks and accomplishments and to appreciate how funny and neurotic and, like most of my friends, stressed-out she was. One night we really opened up to one another—or, rather, opened up our shirts. We'd taken to having pizza every Monday night with our children at her house, while our husbands had one night of freedom. We were talking about the usual subjects mothers discuss—gripes about fatigue and husbands not doing enough and the impossible juggling act of demands—when we landed on the subject of nursing.

Over a guilty glass of white wine, we confessed to one another about days we'd arrived at work so engorged that milk leaked out of our nursing pads and bras and onto our shirts. We swapped stories about how our breasts were often so full that, before we could even start pumping, the milk would spurt out, shooting like uncorked champagne. We'd rarely heard about this phenomenon, and God knows we had never openly talked about it with anyone else. You always hear about projectile vomiting. But why never projectile milking? Within a few minutes we were snorting and crying with laughter. All that hoopla must have startled Sam and Tessa, who'd been dozing in our laps. They started rooting and crying for milk. Like dogs salivating for a bone, our breasts began dripping milk.

It was the ideal opportunity. After such a confessional, we'd shed any shame about our ta-tas. We let loose, willing the milk to not just flow, but gush. We were like sportsmen who excel in an obscure skill such as, say, elephant polo, but can't easily go about demonstrating their mastery to the general public. From where we sat at her dining room table, we both shot several inches away. Our milk landed in a glistening pool on her dining room table, just near the pizza box.

So, who won? Without a referee present, without an official goal to hit, it would have been impossible to prove *exactly*. But, without false pride, I'd like to go on record that I'm almost certain my mighty little breasts outperformed Kirstin's, milk-wise. My shot landed at least a couple of inches farther, making me the Barry Bonds of breast milk. It was great to know that, finally, I'd won.

I'd forgotten that sense of dairy-pride until recently, when I had a second child. I'd taken my first airplane trip with my then two-month-old daughter, Molly, and nine-year-old Sam. Even though I was traveling without my husband, I felt remarkably in control. We had made it onto the plane with a minute or two to spare and located our seats in the kids' ghetto in row 43. Moments after I stuffed the diaper bag under my seat and secured Sam's and my seat belts in place, we had liftoff, and I had let-down.

Molly had gone without milk for nearly two hours, a long time for a newborn. I'd been aching to feed her, and I sensed she was on the edge of despair and about to cry. So I went through some contortions to get her comfortably in place in my small airplane seat and my breast out of my clothing and into her mouth.

Sam, seated to my right, was riveted by his new Game Boy, which he wasn't supposed to turn on until we ascended, but I let him anyway. He jabbed me gently with his elbow and said, "Oh, man! This is sooooo funny, Mom! This is sooooo great. Look at Mario! Look! *Look!*"

I turned to give him my full attention, forgetting that my breast was firmly attached to my body. So there it went, my springy yet engorged left breast, as it popped free from Molly's mouth.

Now everything started happening at once.

Molly was wailing, in that singular, stomach-curdling baby shriek that's ten thousand times worse on a plane. Sam, mysteriously oblivious to her wails, continued to insist I take a really close look at his Game Boy screen. "Mom! *Mo-om!*" I suspected I'd become the most unpopular person on the plane or, for some in the audience, the most popular, given my spontaneous topless show right there in the friendly skies.

That's why, as I look back, it's a surprise to me that I didn't instantly (a) stick my breast back in Molly's mouth or (b) notice that a steady arc of milk was spraying up and over the seat in front of me. I was so preoccupied with all of the chaos that it took more than several seconds for me to realize that the passenger sitting directly in front of me must have been in my breast's line of fire, because he was tapping his hair and looking at his hand. That's when I reattached Molly to my chest, both to stop her crying and to ensure I wasn't implicated.

Since the man was glancing up towards all of the control

buttons above him, I imagined he was probably thinking, "Hmm, weird. My hair is wet. Probably air-conditioning coolant." I'm pretty sure, since he didn't turn around to glare at *yet another woman spraying him with breast milk on the plane,* that he hadn't figured out I was the moisture source.

I was embarrassed, of course. But probably not as much as I should have been. My shame was, to tell the truth, eclipsed by pride. I still had it. After all those years, I remained a sharp-shooter, the mistress of my mammaries. I mean, that was really something, to have shot *that* far and *that* high. Yet, in an act of undisputed Olympian caliber, a success I could never have imagined possible in my lifetime, I was essentially alone to bask in my moment of glory. If only Kirstin, to this day my close friend, were there with me. God, I would have shown her.

✳

Leslie Crawford is a writer living in San Francisco with her husband, Steve, and two children, Sam and Molly. Crawford is a regular contributor to *San Francisco Magazine* and BabyCenter.com, and she has written for *Metropolis, Salon, Garden Design,* and other publications.

IN A MAN'S WORLD

Dawn Porter

After a two-year journey with infertility doctors that culminated in two rounds of in vitro fertilization, I had my first child at the age of thirty-five. That made me a "mature" mother, in the parlance of baby making. I am a lawyer by training, and I like to think I'm the analytical sort, so at first I liked being grouped with a lot of other women, especially since everyone I knew was in the same category. But gradually you have a way of internalizing labels and their meanings, so that in between calculating the risk of serious birth defects, premature labor, preeclampsia, and gestational diabetes, I resolved that if I should be so lucky as to actually produce a healthy baby, I'd make up for having him at such an advanced age.

At the time I was working in New York City for ABC News as the director of standards and practices. My job was to review stories for accuracy and context. In the news business, the credibility of the network is essential (ask Dan Rather). So, in addition to reading our scripts and reviewing screening copies of news stories before they went on air, it was also my job to keep up with current events and reporting by other networks. Or, as my husband says, I was paid to watch television.

And watch I did. During my pregnancy I was comforted by the seemingly endless supply of news stories about companies welcoming nursing mothers back to the workplace. In those hazy days, I entertained myself by looking for attractive maternity clothes at Liz Lange sample sales, and I read and watched everything related to pregnancy. I liked to use my lunch break to walk over to the Upper Breast Side, a store devoted entirely to the needs of nursing mothers. Gazing in rapture alongside the other expectant mothers at the milk-collection bags, I fell hard for the image of me and my fat, happy baby, bonding over a good long drink of "liquid gold." That's what the books call it, *gold*. No pressure or anything. I mean, if I was speaking in Spanish while meditating and playing him classical music for brain development, how could I give him anything but nature's perfect food? My favorite articles were about the juggling acts performed by working mothers: Mothers with lactation rooms and rocking chairs. Mothers who had their nannies bring the babies in to nurse two or more times a day. Mothers who nursed their babies *during* meetings. As if. Armed with all these glowing accounts of women having it all, the reality came as something of a shock. I don't know what kinds of jobs these women have, but I can tell you with confidence that nothing kills conversation faster than whipping out your breast, even if there is a baby nearby. (I later used this tactic quite successfully when I wanted to get some peace and quiet at home.)

I loved my job, and I was extremely proud to be part of ABC News. The corporation was full of smart, hard-working people, most of whom had good intentions and all of whom were ambitious. In 2001, when I had my first child, mothers in the newsroom and the executive offices were no longer a novelty. There were many, many smart, capable women who had had children and come back to work. So many, in fact, that when I was pregnant it didn't occur to me that it would be a novel thing to return to my job *and* continue to nurse my son. Nursing was part of mothering, right? I gave little thought to all the details attendant to breastfeeding as a working mother, issues such as where I would actually use the breast pump, and how long it would take to set it up, get it going, extract the milk, and then clean myself and the pump to my exacting hygienic standards. I thought I'd just figure it out as all those women before me had done.

But, like all fantasies, this one crashed head-on into reality. To say the first nursing was harder than I'd expected is something of an understatement. It would take several excruciating minutes to get that squiggling little baby in what was supposed to be the right position. Then, just when I thought we had it, he'd slide down on the breast and do the dreaded "nipple suck," leaving me with red and raw nipples that cracked and blistered. It also took a *loooong* time to feed the baby, so that by the time he was full and burped, it was nearly time to do it all over again. Instead of the joyous bonding time I'd imagined, feeding him was actually something of a chore. It would be so much faster to give him a nice warm bottle, from which I could see those nice neat ounces disappear. But I'd read all the literature and I was determined to stick with breastfeeding. It was hard. Really hard.

The low point came when the baby was about a week old. I found myself sitting in my living room, naked from the waist up, with my mother holding the baby on one side and my husband cheering on the other as I tried to guide my breast into the baby's open mouth like a 747 coming in for a landing. We managed to get everything in the right place after a good fifteen minutes or so, but this team approach was not exactly a long-term solution. Me naked, mother aiming baby, husband saying, "Open wide," and opening his mouth to show the baby what to do. Um, no. We couldn't continue this way.

We called a lactation consultant, who came with funny tubes and special official-looking bottles and tips about how to make the baby open his little mouth as wide as a striped bass does. I did what lawyers do; I took notes (I still have them somewhere). We kept trying, he and I, and then one day, somehow, magically, we got it. I felt a sharp tug and a stab of not-quite-pain, but something that was "uncomfortable," as they say, but not deadly, and then, lordy, lordy, it looked as if he was doing it. He was sucking, and he was happy. There it was, a baby drinking from my body. No one was more surprised about this development than the baby, who opened his eyes wide in shock when he got a good mouthful of milk from the breast.

After that we fell into something of a rhythm. I never became one of those women who could whip it out and feed the baby while say, driving, but we managed. Always a little worried that he wasn't actually getting any food, I drank fenugreek tea and tons of water and peered into his adorable well-fed eyes, searching for signs of dehydration. In the back of my mind I began to wonder how anyone managed to shower or read mail, let alone return calls or, um, work. Three months stretched to four, then five, and then in hypertime the fall was nearing an end and it was time to return to my job.

I'd bought a pump around the second week of pregnancy (with plenty of storage supplies from the Upper Breast Side), and I was using it at home in preparation for pumping in the office. I even worked out a schedule on paper. It was neat and pretty; I highlighted parts of it.

But, once again, reality was not so neat. First, I'd thought I could pump during The Call, when all the senior producers and reporters tell what news stories they are following during the day and give their preliminary thoughts about what they will pitch to the evening news team for that night's show. I thought this was a splendid idea, since, after all, I was never going to actually *talk* (talking was for a coveted few), and since everyone I worked with would also be listening to The Call, either in person or by telephone. Since no one was likely to call me or come see me during that half-hour, I figured it might be a good time to multi-task. But then a friend told me that she once accidentally forgot to mute her phone during a conference call, and the people on the other end asked her what the whirring noise was. The vision of Peter Jennings and a whole room of television anchors and executives listening to my breast pump gave me pause. I thought I'd better not chance it.

Then I thought, No big deal, I'll just pump one or two times during the day. That, too, had its challenges. As for the actual pumping setup, I was lucky; I had a private office and a door with a lock, so pumping a couple of times a day seemed like a reasonable plan, and it was, at least in theory. But pumping involves your mind as much as your body, and the mind of a nursing mother, conflicted about working in the first place, can be a tricky thing. I had the good fortune to be on the same floor as the president of the news division and his senior management team, although I wasn't a senior manager (I was a mid-level executive at best). Having an office on this floor was great for people watching and for keeping score of just who was spending a lot of time with management, but it also meant that all sorts of famous newsmakers, and just plain famous people, were likely to walk down the hall at any time. Let me tell you, watching the president of Pakistan walk past your office does not spur let-down. Same for Vanessa Williams or Madeleine Albright. It was just too easy to get distracted. What with the people watching and the TVs on in my office and my *job*, it was pretty difficult to find the time to pump some days. I'd be trying to pump and also watch Mel Gibson gab with the gals on *The View*. At other times the phone would ring, and I'd have to decide whether to interrupt a good pumping session to talk to a producer. The problem is, producers think *every* question is urgent. And while you are trying to decide whether to let the call roll over to voice mail, you don't know if the person is on a deadline or in the field with a big problem. And then there was the constant worry that I'd forget to lock the door and someone would walk in, or someone would see through the blinds, or some other humiliating encounter would expose me naked with two breasts drawn out into a zucchini shape and spewing a thin stream of white liquid into a bottle with a tell-tale yellow cap. Eew.

As if that wasn't enough, there is the undeniable fact that offices are set up for work, not extracting or storing containers of breast milk. Many a childless woman at the network happened upon me cleaning funnel-like attachments and tubing in the restroom—inevitably, since I did it two or three times a day, depending on what was going on in the world and how late I had to stay at work. It quickly became clear that, as lucky as I was, I needed a new plan. I needed somewhere more private where I could go and pump before scooting back to work.

Why did I stick with it? Partly because I'm stubborn. I'd worked really hard to be able to nurse, and I wanted to (pardon the expression) milk it. And the truth was, even with all the inconveniences I *liked* nursing and wanted to keep it up. After being away from my son all day, nothing made me feel more needed and connected to him than nursing. When he latched on, it was as if he were saying, "Oh! I remember you! I know these breasts! You are my mother! Welcome home."

So I attacked the pumping problem with newfound determination. If people could figure out how nuclear material was shipped in a container across the ocean, I could figure out how to pump at work. Two women I'd become friendly with had had babies around the same time, and when we'd see each other in the halls or the cafeteria we'd compare notes. They were also trying to pump in their offices, with varying degrees of success. One was sharing her office; while I don't think she was shy, this was awkward. Plus people were always barging in. The other had a large and picturesque corner office, but she just couldn't get a lot of milk. She'd pump for what probably felt like hours and would end up with two ounces. This, let me tell you, is the single most depressing thing that can happen to a pumper. You're giving it your all, and your body is just not cooperating.

Looking back on it, I wonder now why we never thought to go to someone in management and ask for a dedicated room for pumping. It wasn't as if management was hostile or anything; we just didn't think to ask, and they didn't offer, and that was that. When I think about it, it does strike me as odd. If a company that employs some of the most powerful women in the world doesn't make it easy for working mothers to continue to nurse, what hope is there for women working in retail or fast food?

One thing you have to give news producers credit for is

that they are extremely resourceful. So one day my friend told me to meet her on her floor because she had found a solution to the pumping problem. We could use the office of a producer who was on the road a lot. My friend had gotten a sympathetic manager to put a dorm-style refrigerator in the office, and there was a couch and several outlets. We were high-fiving like football players. The setup was sweet. The best thing about the room was that somehow the producer *was never there*. Ever. (I still want to know how to get that job.) His cushy setup meant that we could leave the pumps in the office all the time and just head down when we needed to pump.

The pumping went a lot better after that. Word spread about the pumping room, and it became kind of a girls' club. A bunch of people were even sharing a pump that had been used by news producers and on-air talent before them at *World News Tonight*. It became the World News Pump. It was one of those hospital-grade pumps that look like old-style Hoover canister vacuums. I'm a little squeamish, and I found it a bit frightening. But my friend was a real pro. She could hook up both breasts to the pump and, voilà, hands free! I once saw her do hands-free double pumping while talking to a reporter in the field about a story. She was completely unfazed that a machine was sucking on both her breasts while she negotiated language on a piece for the evening news.

One day while my friend was pumping, she reached into the desk drawer to find a pen. Instead of a pen she pulled out a bunch of porno magazines. I don't think they were there for research. We cracked up. We thought it was hilarious that the office of a guy who clearly enjoyed looking at women's naked breasts was now full of naked breasts on a daily basis.

Strangely enough, I never even *met* the producer whose

office we were squatting in, and to this day I don't know if he knew how he'd helped all us pumpers.

I never quite got the hands-free thing down, but the time we used the room was the best I had as a nursing working mother. At some point pumping became too time-consuming, and I wasn't getting enough milk, so I reluctantly gave it up. I think now I should have pressed on a bit longer. I was never a natural at nursing, and it never came easily, but I knew fully and completely that the struggle was worth it. I look at my son these days, full of confidence and able to choose his own food, and I wonder if some part of him remembers the times when it was just the two of us, usually late at night, awake while the house was still and quiet. He'd focus on eating, and I'd focus on him. I marveled at the idea that a substance from my body could nourish his. Nursing was good. Good for the baby. Good for me.

❉

Dawn Porter is now vice president of standards and practices at the A&E Television Networks and is also at work on a biography of nineteenth-century African American suffragist Ida Wells-Barnett. Porter and her husband, David Graff, live in Montclair, New Jersey, with their two sons.

SUBJECT: PUMPING

Nancy M. Williams

At thirty-eight, with a baby daughter and a son in preschool, I negotiated a part-time marketing job at Virgin Mobile USA, a hip, youthful company. Having once built a multimillion-dollar business from a speck of revenue, I now huddled in a cube, executing mundane sales programs. For this depressing state of affairs I blamed my breasts. Not the perky breasts I'd sported B.C. (before children) but rather my new-mother breasts, that uneven, mole-spotted, milk-dribbling duo.

Before children, my marketing career at AT&T had charted a promising arc. A specialist in bringing new products to market, I was adept at conceptualizing strategy and mobilizing large working teams. I savored my reputation as an up-and-comer. I had a staff of five marketing managers, a dedicated secretary, and a spacious office with a pair of meandering philodendrons. The work whirlwind and my crammed calendar invigorated me. Most important, when I spoke, everyone listened.

Motherhood had changed my priorities (although perhaps not my ambitions). I wanted to breastfeed Gracie for at least a year, with as few bottles as possible. Charlie, my son, was reeling from the explosion of his sister's birth and needed my calming presence. My schedule at Virgin Mobile—twenty hours a week, mornings—meant I missed only two feedings with Gracie and could spend the afternoons with my children. During my half-day absences, Charlie and Gracie were well cared for by our neighbor and my husband, David, who ran a business from our home.

My MBA gal pals exclaimed over the situation I'd snared: *So great you can keep on breastfeeding! So cool you're working in a start-up!* I nodded, numbly. In exchange for my seemingly ideal arrangement, I was a cube-squatting, slow-track, part-time loser. I longed for my glory days at AT&T, when I strode onto the executive suite's thick carpet for meetings. Nowadays, the only place I zoomed was to the ladies' room to extract breast milk. *This isn't really me,* I often reassured myself. Yet it was my life; I was scrolling through a chapter I would never have imagined.

That is, until I received an unexpected email from Richard Branson. *Sir* Richard Branson, the billionaire, charismatic entrepreneur who owned Virgin Mobile USA along with four hundred other companies.

The day my inbox trumpeted an email from Sir Richard began like many others. The strap of my black leather nursing bag—laden with hand pump, milk bottles, and spare nursing pads—dug into my shoulder. My briefcase and cooler for pumped milk bumped against my opposite thigh. I hurried past wall posters of cavorting teenaged models, each clutching a Virgin Mobile cell phone. Into my cube's cabinet I stuffed nursing bag and cooler. I didn't like having my pumping paraphernalia on view.

"Yo," said my cubicle neighbor, one of the preppy recent graduates in sales who affected ghetto talk as a way of tapping our youth market's inner soul. He strutted across the hallway in striated indigo jeans.

I complimented his attire, then asked for the document he'd owed me for a week.

"My bad. I'll get that to you"—he flipped open his cell phone, consulting his calendar—"in an hour?"

"Don't forget."

I grimaced. I sounded so almost-fortyish, so teetering on the brink of middle age, so maternal. It wasn't difficult to sound dated at Virgin Mobile. The company was disproportionately populated by single male twenty-somethings who instant-messaged their buddies obsessively, even during meetings. As a nursing mother, I was clearly the odd woman out.

I logged on to my laptop. A handful of new emails roosted in my inbox. I scanned the names of the senders. The third one down was Richard Branson. Was this a joke? No, the email was legit. I stared at his electronic signature: Richard.

A week before, I'd composed, on behalf of a few Virgin Mobile executives, an email about sales strategy bound for Sir Richard. At the bottom I tucked a bulleted, two-line brainstorming idea. Our teen customer base skewed female. Our logo's luscious, deep red evoked lip gloss, and teen girls prowled makeup aisles. My conclusion: We could profit from a partnership with a beauty company.

Richard (we were now on a first-name basis) wrote to say he liked my thinking. He had plucked my idea from the hundreds of daily missives he no doubt received from his diligent executives around the globe. His email granted me permission to forge ahead. I would locate a chic beauty company to burnish the Virgin Mobile brand. Revenue from the alliance would grow until it exploded like a glittering firework. A couple of years from now, when searching for a seasoned marketer to lead his next venture, Richard would tap me. As I considered this delicious fantasy, I leaned back in my ergonomic office chair. I could fall into a soothing sleep.

My Outlook calendar pinged a grating, two-toned reminder. The appointment details flashed onto the screen: *Subject— Pumping; Location—Handicapped Stall.* I had a meeting with my-self in the women's bathroom. Time to pump.

In the ladies' room, warm water sluiced through my fingers and danced down the drain. With Richard's email glowing in my inbox, the risk of invisible organisms swarming through the air and contaminating the milk seemed, for once, remote. I opened the handicapped stall with a clean paper towel gripped between my fingers. Looping one strap of my black bag on the closed door's hook, I removed the hand pump, a plastic bottle already screwed in place.

I pumped standing. Pinning my shirt's hem with my chin (the casual dress code was a boon for nursing mothers), I un-hooked my bra's right side and clamped the suction cup over my breast. I gave a long pull on the handle. Cream-colored milk squirted into the metered plastic bottle. The frothy liquid rose to the one-ounce mark, then the two-ounce mark, while the hand pump swished and clicked its familiar rhythm. At four ounces, an endorphin-induced bliss settled over me, like a gossamer blanket from the breastfeeding fairy.

No matter how stressful my days or sleepless my nights, my breasts produced an abundance of milk. When Charlie was born, he latched on with a textbook-perfect fish mouth. My son gradually tapered his feedings to one nightly nursing, until I weaned him at twenty-one months. Breastfeeding was some-thing I was good at, proof I could be a good mother.

Back at my desk, eight ounces of precious milk stowed inside the cooler, I retrieved Richard's email, gleaming in my inbox like a jewel. Hands shaking, I crafted a short reply, copying my chain of command, including my boss's boss, Howard, a fresh arrival from the music industry and our new marketing chief. Within a few hours of my clicking Send, the entire company knew Richard had pinged me.

"Yo," boomed one of the sales guys. "What's up with the Branson email?"

Howard stopped by my desk. He wore a buzz haircut, a cerulean-blue shirt with black netted pockets, and combat-style khaki pants.

"Slick work with Richard," he said. "Call Donna and get on my calendar."

"Absolutely."

"Cool."

Two weeks later, Howard and I met to review the six cosmetics firms I had selected as partnership finalists. Howard zeroed in on an established door-to-door beauty company. He asked me to assemble a formal proposal.

As I conferred with Supply Chain, Finance, and Advertising to hash out the proposal details, I buzzed with a purposeful joy. I sprinted down hallways to meetings. My vigorous workday spun silk strands, tossing the connecting threads to the self of my twenties and early thirties. As for pumping, my twice-daily appointments in the handicapped stall became an annoying obligation I squeezed in between meetings.

The night before a large team session, I worked late in my attic study. David stomped up the stairs.

"You're putting too much time into this project. And you're not being compensated for it."

"This is an investment in my career!"

David rolled his eyes to the slanted ceiling. "You don't need this on your resumé. Believe me, it's impressive enough."

"That's old stuff. I need something new."

"Sleep. That's what you need."

The next morning swirled with phone calls, emails, instant messages. I skipped my first pumping appointment, resolving to glean extra ounces during lunch. But when my calendar shot out its reminder (*Subject—Pumping; Location—Handicapped Stall*) my Supply Chain contact huffed over: His boss was waffling about the large quantity of phones required for the beauty deal.

To handle this "fire drill," I would skip pumping.

A conscientious voice, the one that had choked and almost drowned in the Branson-email tidal wave, regained its strength and chastened me. *You're going to mess up your breastfeeding schedule. Keep this up, and soon you won't have enough milk.*

I don't care, the leadership-hungry part of my self retorted. I flounced, with more bravado than Scarlett O'Hara at the Wilkeses' mansion picnic, to an emergency lunchtime session, during which I convinced the Supply Chain VP to set aside enough phones.

I had one minute to scramble to my team meeting. As I streaked across the floor, I realized I had neglected to tell David I would be late. Patting my pockets for my cell phone, I visualized it on the kitchen counter, where I'd left it that morning in my rush to leave. I was already late for the meeting. David would figure it out.

At the conference room door, I stopped. Fifteen people sat at the table. They had left one empty chair at the head. That seat was for me. Early-afternoon sunlight slanted through the cracked blinds and ignited my chair's chrome trim. A thin coating of white light, like smooth ice, pooled on the oval conference table. Five years had passed since I had conducted a session of this scope. The prospect dazzled me.

My breasts chose that moment to balk. They pressed into my rib cage and bulged against my nursing bra. I decided, as I took my seat and described the agenda, to ignore them. What did they know, that ornery, complaining twosome, encased in a milk-stained nursing bra?

As the team checked off the agenda's first issue, then discussed the second, worry seeped inside me until it coursed like a submerged stream. What if, in the middle of this meeting, my throbbing breasts gushed a leak? My right breast, the smaller of the pair B.C., could become especially engorged, the nipple thrust to the side, the tissue rigid and bumpy from gummed milk ducts. I hunched forward, hoping no one would notice my uneven chest.

As we reviewed the third and final question, I imagined Gracie's pout with protruding lower lip ballooning to a full cry, her rosy skin deepening to an outraged red, her little hands clenched in protesting fists. My baby could be crying right now. As much as I rejoiced and exulted in this chair, as much as presiding over this meeting reminded me of my old self, did I need to be that person right now? I had vowed not to be her, at least until I weaned Gracie.

Meeting over, proposal points wrapped up, my breasts sparing me a mortifying leak, I careened through the parking lot. During the half-hour drive home, I agonized whether to exit the freeway to call David.

On the porch I fumbled in my briefcase for the house key. David yanked open the kitchen door. In his arms sat Gracie, her plump cheeks glistening, her eyes beseeching, her voice whimpering. I knew that pleading cry, one I prided myself on rarely hearing from my children. She had screamed for too long and was now spent with exhaustion. She was very, very hungry.

"Where were you?" David asked.

"I'm sorry." I lifted Gracie from his arms and made a beeline for my breastfeeding spot on the living room couch.

David followed. "Why didn't you call? I held off giving her a bottle."

I didn't reply. I wanted to avoid a fight with David and distance myself from the person who had treated her baby so carelessly. Balancing Gracie on my nursing pillow, I peeled away my bra's right flap. Gracie latched on hard, pulling out the milk with a hungry gulp.

David shook his head. "That was so irresponsible."

"I know," I said.

The pressure deflated, not only in my milk ducts but also in my throbbing head, as Gracie sucked out the milk. Her warm hand wandered past my collarbone to grab a fistful of hair. She liked to hold on while nursing. I traced the outline of her apricot ear.

For the next few days, I cringed whenever I remembered stressing my baby. I didn't want to endanger my ability to breastfeed Gracie. Yet I still harbored my old self, the thirty-year-old with unmarked breasts and confidence in her ability to succeed. I had coveted that head chair at the conference table because I couldn't relinquish a cherished part of myself. From the standpoint of the leader inside, my breasts had shackled me.

As much as returning to my insignificant, diminished work self pained me, the possibility of Gracie's weaning early hurt far more. I had to choose, not in an ambivalent way, but clearly and decisively. The following Monday, I asked Howard to remove me from the beauty project.

He nodded thoughtfully. "So you'll incubate ideas, then let an operational team take them to market?"

"Yes, that would be good."

"Cool."

Not completely cool. Resigned, I slunk to my desk and turned on my laptop. I looped the cursor around the screen in wide, aimless circles.

In my mind I heard the voices of two friends, a married couple with older children. They had counseled, as though the matter were zipped up, that parenthood was about making choices. At the time, their advice had made me uncomfortable. Now I understood why. My friends, although experienced parents, failed to describe the sometimes visceral process of making choices. They skipped over the messy struggle. They omitted mention of chiseling cuts, the marble shards of desires left behind.

I sat up in my chair. I created an electronic folder and deposited inside Sir Richard Branson's email endorsing the beauty project. This folder, christened Branson, would be visible each time I opened my inbox. I would keep it on hand, and occasionally review its contents, as a reminder of the person that I had chosen, at this time in my life, not to be.

❊

Nancy M. Williams led Virgin Mobile USA's e-commerce sales and marketing group until late 2006, when she took a sabbatical from her marketing career to focus on creative writing. Her work has appeared in *Fit Pregnancy* and *New Jersey Family* magazines. She lives in Montclair, New Jersey, with her husband, David, and her two children.

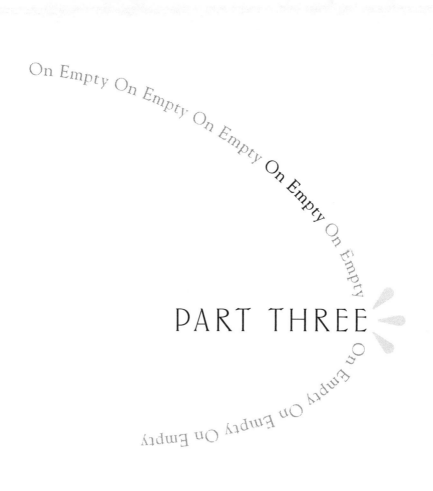

On Empty On Empty On Empty On Empty On Empty On Empty

PART THREE

On Empty On Empty On Empty

ANATHEMA MOM

Alice Elliott Dark

It happens again. A casual discussion among a group of women becomes personal and revealing. Sorrows and frustrations are shared, private narratives are unfurled, and confessions are made, based on an assumption that we share common experiences and views. We tell our stories and receive in return a warm, galvanizing thrill of revelation and acceptance. Bearing and raising these children is magical, but it is also hard—harder than we ever imagined when our mothers were doing it all wrong. It's a relief to have moments when we can talk about it. A lot of the time, when we're alone in the house with the kids and deeply exhausted or frustrated, it feels as though no one else could possibly feel as angry or victimized or as much like running away as we do. Conversation isn't hard to come by, especially not about childbirth. We can plop down next to a complete stranger and speak intimately about blood, pain, and glory. Men with their sports have nothing on us—except sports bars. There are no childbirth bars, but never mind. We have doctors' offices, playgrounds, Starbucks. We get by.

Today I'm among women I know, but our war stories are new

to each other. From time to time I like to tell mine—the head-line is a grabber. My obstetrician is in jail, I say. All heads turn to-wards me, and I have the floor for several minutes. He's in prison, not because of me, although I could have sued him. Listen to this—he cranked up the dial on my Pitocin drip so high that the nurse screamed, *You are killing this woman!* My husband cried. My labor failed to advance. After forty-eight hours, I had a c-section.

I have more to tell about this, but my turn is over. That's okay—it felt good to retell even this small part of it. Repetition pushes it further into the past.

The talk rambles, climbs hills, settles in verdant valleys. This is an adult lullaby, this chatter among women. We're talk-ing about something mythological in its power. How freaky is it, really, that we can grow another human being inside our own bodies? We can be ultimately creative while still per-forming our daily tasks. We are incredible. We are miraculous. You can't make this stuff up!

I'm part of the secret; I'm enjoying myself, listening, em-pathizing. Then a voice rings out, strong and clear, full of con-viction. A proclamation is made: *That's why it's so important to breastfeed.*

I agree. How could I not? The advice is ubiquitous, imparted even during commercials for formula. We all know. Breast is best.

The breastfeeding war stories begin. I am silent. I have nothing to add to this conversation. I don't know what it feels like, I don't know about leaking at embarrassing times, or how sexual the sensation is, or about mastitis, or about my boobs shrinking, or having the baby weight sucked off of me. I didn't breastfeed. I don't want to say this, either, because it inevitably leads to a series of prosecutorial questions, at the end of which I'm reassured, or placated—if I'm among nice people—that it doesn't matter. No one believes this, though, and the spell of mutuality is broken. I messed up.

*   *

It's sixteen years earlier, and I'm in Lenox Hill Hospital, in the neonatal intensive care unit. This is not a peaceful place. All around me machines are beeping and wheezing, lights blaze, nurses squeak past briskly. I've fought with a few of them already over my right to read my baby's chart—I'm paying for what is written there, aren't I?—and my insistence that they let me feed him. I need to get the feeding going, he needs my early milk, he needs to learn and so do I. I took baby classes, I've read about this. I know.

I am rebuffed on all counts. No. No and no and no. None of this is about me. It's about nurses and babies and machines. I am . . . in the way.

So a few days into his incarceration, I stand uselessly by his incubator, watching him breathe. The charge against him is that he wasn't breathing correctly twenty-four hours into life. He is being held without trial, intermittently observed. His only nourishment is an intravenous drip, and he's losing weight fast.

A nurse passes by. "Can't he have a pacifier, please? He needs to learn how to suck."

"I'll have to ask the doctor."

"When will he—or she—be here?"

"It's the weekend. He doesn't do regular rounds on the weekend."

"There must be a doctor here who could authorize a pacifier."

"When someone comes, I'll ask."

"Ask for a bottle. He's doing fine, isn't he?"

She glances at his chart. "His bilirubin is high."

"But his breathing is fine, right? So he could have a bottle, or I could start breastfeeding?"

"Maybe." She isn't looking at me.

"When can he leave?"

"Not until after the weekend, at the earliest. We have no one to authorize signing babies out on the weekend."

"The someone who is coming can't authorize that?"

No answer.

"But he shouldn't be in here in the first place! My obstetrician said there's nothing wrong with him!"

This was true. He'd looked in on the baby several times. I didn't know then that no one believed a thing that came out of that guy's mouth.

She glares at me. I can tell she wants to slap me. The feeling is mutual. She has a job to keep, however, and I'm certainly not the only hysterical woman she's seen in that awful place. We fume at each other.

"I'll ask," she says finally. Squeak, squeak, she zooms off.

I can feel my incision oozing. Against all my desires, I trudge back to my room, miles away, holding my IV pole instead of my baby.

※　※

I pump. My five days of paid hospitalization are up and I have to leave—without my baby. I pump. I pump. I'm alone in my bed in my apartment, trying to recover from the ripped incision. I am calm. I am crazy. Did I really have a baby? I can't believe it—I mean I really can't. I think I was dreaming. I know

I was pregnant, I loved being pregnant, I had a relationship with the fetus, we named him at twenty weeks when we learned a boy was coming to us. He'd been Asher to me for four months before he was born. Asher was my baby. But was he really the same as the tiny creature over in the Lenox Hill NICU? That baby was so . . . unfamiliar. Asher was active and lively. The baby in the plastic incubator looked like a chicken in a roasting pan. Maybe he was switched with my real baby. Maybe my baby hadn't been born yet after all, and he was still resting quietly inside me. Maybe I was never pregnant and I was still my old self who I'd been for the thirty-eight previous years.

I pump. There's not much coming. I'm reading about breastfeeding and nothing is happening the way it says in the books. I don't have what is called let-down. I'm not spurting milk. My breasts aren't huge. I get a little bit out each time, maybe an ounce. That's it.

I call a woman who bills herself as a "lactation expert." I'm desperate enough to get past such a cumbersome term if she can help me. She tells me not to worry, that the baby will stimulate me; all will be well when he comes home.

The pump makes its weird squelchy noise that makes me think of walking in the mud. I hand my husband the nearly empty beakers of milk I produce, and he throws them out. The nurses still aren't feeding the baby, so the milk is useless. I'm in too much pain to go visit him. I can hardly even walk to the bathroom. My husband goes to the hospital and comes back with reports. We are living in limbo. If you ask me who I am, I won't have a good answer.

I am both numb and in pain. That's all I know.

*   *

It's a couple of days later and I'm going nuts. We ask a top Upper East Side pediatrician to go look at the baby and she says he's absolutely fine. My mother says all her babies were yellow with bilirubin; you just put them by the window and it goes away. I decide keeping babies prisoner because of a high bilirubin count is a new way for hospitals to make money. I'm going to research this! Write an article about it!

I am comforting myself with familiar ways of controlling information. I'm deflecting grief. Or trying to. It's not working.

Finally my husband and a friend who has a job that comes with a badge go take the baby. On a Sunday night, they walk into the NICU, they pick him up, and they take him. The nurses try to stop them, but his friend flashes the badge and my husband says, *You'll have to arrest me to stop me*.

They bring Asher home, and my new life begins.

✳   ✳

The lactation expert stands beside the bed. She's large and earth-motherly; she'd have surely been a wet nurse in another era. We're trying, hard. My breasts are exposed, the expert pours warm milk over them for the baby to catch in his mouth, but he is crying. Every so often there's a moment when he seems to grab my nipple but soon his jaw goes slack and the nipple hangs there, useless. I do everything the woman tells me, everything I have read in books, but none of it is working. The baby isn't latching on. Isn't sucking. Isn't getting anything.

I have been supplementing with a bottle—and a very tiny bottle it is, almost like the kind you feed a kitten with—because he's so thin it frightens me. He was born at six pounds but weighed only five when he came home. The pediatrician wants him to put on weight. I want him to put on weight. It's hard to imagine how he's going to go from being this tiny bag of bones to being one of those round, laughing babies you can cuddle. I'm nearly afraid to hold him now, and I can't bear to bathe him. This is all wrong.

The expert tells me I'm interfering with the process by supplementing, that he's never going to learn unless I stick to the breast and stop the supplementation. When he's hungry enough he'll figure it out.

He cries all the time. His cries shoot straight forward from his lungs—projectile wails. They pierce me in soft spots. I can go on only by telling myself one hundred times an hour that this is for the best. I don't believe it.

The lactation expert comes back a few more times. She's a high-energy coach, full of cheers and coaxes for the baby and me, but nothing is happening. She can't understand it. Skepticism comes into her eyes as she looks at me. Am I supplementing? I assure her I'm not, but I can see she doesn't believe me. She's preparing to write me off. The failure is mine and mine alone. Sure enough, when it's time to make another appointment, she says she's taught me all she knows and that I just have to keep trying. She takes her check and scrams.

Asher can't sleep for very long because he's hungry. He can't drink more than an ounce at a time. His weight drops. I don't need a scale to tell me that. I can see it.

I am so exhausted I can't even hold him. I fall into a dead sleep. When I awake my husband says he gave the baby a bottle, and the baby drank an ounce. I don't know how to feel about this. I want the baby to eat, but I want to be the one to feed him. BREAST IS BEST! The words run through my mind in huge letters, like skywriting. I can't stop weeping.

*   *

It begins with a fever. Soon my entire abdomen is in pain. I'm dying for real now, I know it.

I call my obstetrician. He's good for saying, *Come right in.* He saved my baby this way twice during the pregnancy. He is years away from jail, and I still think he's something of a genius, if unorthodox. I need him, and in my need I forgive.

He examines me and runs some tests. I lie there for hours.

"Puerperal fever," he says, with the glee of a man in control of some prize information.

I've never heard of it.

"Childbed fever."

He has to be kidding.

"Not dangerous anymore. You take the Flagyl for three weeks, you'll be fine." He pats me reassuringly, which I like, but he isn't taking any responsibility, which I don't admire at all. Shouldn't he be? I thought unwashed hands, anaerobic bacteria, caused childbed fever. Wouldn't that be his fault?

Long story short: It turns out that while he was doing the c-section he also cut out three enormous fibroids—thereby doing me a favor, he says. *Maybe there was too much trauma to the uterus*, he conjectures. He's more curious than guilty.

Oh.

"I'm breastfeeding," I say—though it's not strictly true. But it is my true intention.

"You throw out all the milk. This medicine is poison to the baby. You pump for three weeks and throw it all out. Then we test your milk and see."

"See what?"

"If it is safe."

*　*

Why can't I get the pump to work? I've heard so many stories of women pumping between meetings in corporate offices, having their breasts squirt the instant they see the pump, pumping so much that the icebox is full and they have to toss some down the drain.

I can barely achieve any milk at all, much less throw away abundance. An ounce or two at each occasion, and it takes about an hour.

My baby is feeding every two hours or so, sometimes more often.

I am so exhausted I can't . . . I can't even . . .

I can't go on.

*　*

It's over. The decision is made. No breast.

First a c-section, now this. My baby can barely suck, but I do, big time.

I suck as a mother already. Just as I feared I would.

I'm so disappointed I can hardly breathe.

*　*

I read an article that cheers me.

Breast milk is good, yes. Nutritionally, it has advantages. But for brain development, it is the stimulation of contact with the mother that is of benefit. Bottle-fed babies who are spoken to, looked at in the eye, stroked, jostled, sung to, develop IQs as high as breastfed babies. It's the communication that counts.

Finally, I have done something right. I look at Asher, always. We play games while he eats. We connect as best we can, with a hunk of plastic between us.

We'll be okay. Or so says the article. I clip it out and put it in my bag. There will come a moment when I'll want to whip it out. If only to bolster me.

*   *

Scene in park.

I'm sitting on a bench with Asher in my lap. He's been running around for a while and is hungry now. He's about thirteen months.

There are several women sitting near me. They know each other and are chatting as they feed their babies. I see them look over at me. I wouldn't mind joining in the conversation. Following a toddler around a playground is mind-numbing as far as I'm concerned. It's cinchy to meet other mothers in New York. I'm up for it.

They look over at me and we all smile. Then they look at Asher. The mood changes.

Stranger: "You feed your baby with a bottle?"

Me: "Yup."

Stranger: "But it's your milk, right?"

"No, it's formula."

"Breast milk is better," she informs me.

"I can't breastfeed."

"Everyone can breastfeed. Have you called La Leche? Their whole point is that there's no such thing as a woman who can't breastfeed. You just have to be committed to it."

"I was committed to it. It didn't work out for me."

"Why? What happened?"

She's judgmental before she even knows my circumstances—but then, so are many other women of my generation. What is wrong with these mothers? Where's the motherliness? Have they got no compassion to spare for the likes of me?

I am still exhausted, I have undiagnosed postpartum depression, my understanding of the events surrounding my son's birth hasn't come yet—so I try to explain. I defend myself, weakly, as I judge myself, too. Stranger listens skeptically, presses me for details, as if eager to catch me in a lie. When she is finished with me, I am thoroughly depressed.

"You could try again, you know," she says. "Lactation can be stimulated at any time. Even men have been known to breastfeed with proper stimulation."

Oh. Well. That nails my coffin shut. I'm not even the mother a man can be.

I wish I had had in my arsenal then the weapon I have since been given by my best friend. Here's what to say when you are attacked like this: *Excuse me, but did I sleep with you last night? Because if I didn't, you have no right to speak to me about my child.*

We go our separate ways. Too late, I think of showing her my article. I realize, though, that she wouldn't believe it. No one will. I throw it in a trash basket on my way home.

* *

Multiply that scene by a hundred. That's what it is like to bottle-feed a baby in a breastfeeding world. I was essentially an abuser—robbing my child of nutrition and the possibility of a full life.

Rooms got quiet when I pulled out the bottle. For years.

I worried, a lot, about whether formula was really enough.

I cringed every time there was an article in the paper about what an infant gets from breast milk in the first three weeks of life. It always sounds like health insurance—the equivalent of receiving a $10 million trust fund at birth. If you get that early milk, you have no worries ahead of you.

How about all the articles about greedy multinationals dumping formula on Africa, tricking tribal women into plying their children with inferior nutrition?

When you are a failure at something, your defeat is pointed out to you in many ways.

It hurts.

*　　*

The conversation goes on around me. Suddenly I surprise myself.

"I didn't breastfeed," I announce.

There's the usual silence.

"I wanted to. I wanted to very badly. But I couldn't."

I see a woman, a friend, lean forward, getting ready to begin the questions.

I'm not going to answer them anymore.

"I have to ask you to trust and believe me about this. I couldn't breastfeed. Asher drank formula, almost exclusively, for three years. He was underweight and ate sparsely, so it was important to make sure he had enough calories every day. He's sixteen now, taller than I am, and healthy. He never gets colds. He scores in high percentiles on standardized tests. He's okay. Breast might be best, but it's not the only answer. I'm really, really tired of the assumption that just because I'm a certain kind of educated, progressive-minded person I breastfed, too. I didn't. I was ashamed of that for a long time, but I can't be anymore."

The women nod. They heard me, it seems—or some of them did. I hope so. In any case, I spoke.

❊

Alice Elliott Dark is the author of the novel *Think of England* and two collections of short stories, *In the Gloaming* and *Naked to the Waist*. She is the writer in residence of the English Department at Rutgers-Newark.

BECAUSE I DON'T WANT TO

Patricia Berry

I did not breastfeed. I have three beautiful daughters who were fed solely on Enfamil from the day each was born until she was about a year old.

There was nothing wrong with them at their births. No incubators separated us. No sucking mechanisms malfunctioned in their altogether perfect little mouths. Nor was there a medical reason I couldn't nurse. My mammary glands appeared to be in working order. Milk engorged me within hours of each delivery, and my infants' cries triggered a sensation that would occur over and over—long past the time my milk had dried up, for years, in fact—that feeling of a hundred little needles pricking at my breasts. But I didn't answer the summons.

Even so, I fit the breastfeeder demographic to a T: older (I was thirty-two when my first was born), college-educated (check), middle-class (yes), and able to stay home with my children (I stopped working full time a year after my second child was born). Almost all of my friends—college classmates, colleagues, childhood pals—nursed their babies, even the ones who didn't have particularly warm and fuzzy feelings about it.

It was what you did. So why on those birth days, my breasts swollen to enormous proportions, was I wrestling into sports bras one size too small in order to squelch milk production?

Was it modesty? I am definitely not the type of woman who can whip it out anytime, anyplace. But had it been my intention to feed my infants by the breast, I would have found a way to do so on my own prudish terms.

Convenience? Let's just say even I can't rationalize how unbuttoning my pajama top could be more complicated than fumbling in the middle of the night with a roll of plastic Playtex bottle liners. Not to mention the inconvenience to our bank account of funding formula and bottles, outlays for three babies for a year that had to total $5,000. To my way of thinking, these expenses were as necessary as the car seat and stroller.

Some irrational fear of—what? Toxic breast milk? I'm a strapping, healthy woman. I don't smoke, I'm not a big drinker, and I wasn't on medication. I've read that lactating women carry minuscule amounts of all kinds of nasty substances in their milk—PCBs, paint thinners, insect poisons—but I would have been astonished to learn mine was anything but 100 percent Grade A.

I could give you some line like "My mother didn't love me enough," but that would be (a) untrue and (b) a cop-out. My mother loved (and still loves) me as most mothers do: in the best way she knew how. And, like many other mothers in the 1950s and 1960s, Mom was encouraged by her pediatrician to feed us, my brother and me, by the bottle.

I, however, had something she didn't: scientific proof that breast milk is best. Moms today know what our mothers might have suspected, even though their doctors often told them otherwise: Ounce for ounce, the fats, nutrients, and disease-fighting substances in breast milk trump formula. If I was to love my children in the best way *I* knew how, I would breastfeed them, right?

Frankly, the notion of suckling my child—the very word *suckling*—made my skin crawl (the feeling we called heebie-jeebies as kids). I could not imagine, let alone imagine *enjoying*, an infant slurping milk through my nipples without quivering with uneasiness. I can tolerate discomfort. I've run marathons despite blisters the size of kumquats, for goodness' sake. But the anxiety produced by the very thought of—forgive me—sucking it up and trying just once for my baby's sake to feed by the breast was more than I could handle. Friends have asked if I associated my breasts with sex, a connection that might explain my aversion. I guess it's possible, but I doubt it. I just couldn't get past that image of a slurping baby. It made me . . . queasy.

I understood that it was a selfish choice. But my mind was made up long before I was ever pregnant. I would weather the storm of disapproval I fully expected to meet. Besides, it was no one else's business.

What I didn't anticipate was that disapproval would hit close to home. Very close. So absolutely clearheaded was I about not breastfeeding that it hadn't occurred to me my husband might feel differently. To this day I rely on Mitch's even temper and levelheadedness. His approval matters to me. Breastfeeding wasn't something we even discussed until I was pregnant with my oldest daughter. Nor do I recall our earliest conversation on the subject.

One evening stands out, though. We both worked long hours, and we'd save bedtime for catching up. But pillow talk turned edgy one night. Mitch, who knew by then I didn't want to breastfeed, asked whether I'd rethought my decision. (He knew better than to come right out and make his case.) I hadn't.

I don't recall his next words exactly, only that he chose them carefully. "What do you think it is that's making you feel this way?"

My throat tightened, a reaction to the disapproval he barely attempted to hide. "I don't know," I managed to squeeze out. "I just don't want to."

He waited.

"The whole idea of it just . . . grosses me out." There, I said it. Surely we could close the door on the subject.

More silence. "That's unusual, isn't it?"

"It's how I feel."

"But how could you not at least *try*?"

The frustration in his voice was palpable. To him my decision was inconceivable.

"I just can't."

"That's not good enough."

"It's good enough for me," I said tearfully, angry for being pressed into a corner but knowing he was right.

He gave up and quickly fell asleep. (How do men do that?) I rolled over on my side and wept. As if my hormones weren't wreaking enough havoc with my emotions, Mitch's disappointment made me miserable. Eventually I slipped downstairs and wrapped myself in a blanket on the couch, feeling huge and sorry for myself. *How could I not?* It was an utterly unmaternal instinct. And yet I knew to my very core I wasn't going to breastfeed. He didn't have to like it, but couldn't he just accept it? My girlfriends understood; why couldn't my *best* friend?

In fairness to Mitch, I don't think the subject came up all that often. It's not as though he berated me daily for my selfishness. Maybe five or six times during my first pregnancy the topic would get heated enough to bring tears—mine mostly. It hung there, though, a small cloud and a bitter aside to the overall excitement we felt over the pending arrival of our first child.

Was it possible I didn't really want children? I didn't think so, although Mitch was ready for kids before I was. Finding Mitch filled me. Here was a good man, a smart, funny, and perfectly imperfect man who tolerated my untidiness and made me feel safe and loved, a man destined to be a great father. But what was the rush?

Once I became pregnant, I rolled through monthly doctor's appointments, baby preparations, and showers while working full time. But I didn't bask in the glow of pregnancy. Always tall, I was the size of a small garage by eight months. I waddled along, though, comforted by the knowledge that this wouldn't last forever, looking forward to running and eating sushi again, relieved that I was over whatever it was that kept me from wanting to start a family.

We had fun planning. Picking names could fill an evening. We narrowed our choices to Malcolm for a boy, Fiona for a girl. And then my cousin came for dinner. *Fiona?* His peas flew in a spit-take across our dining room table, and then he laughed uncontrollably. Mitch and I looked at each other wide-eyed as pride in our originality flitted away. Not one of our daughters is named Fiona.

On the breastfeeding front, I interviewed the pediatrician I'd selected to be sure she wasn't going to hound me on the subject. (She wasn't.) I did not look forward to telling my mother-in-law, but as it turned out Laney was my most ardent supporter. She called often, at work and at home, to check in. Laney saw nothing wrong with my bottle-feeding plan, or if she did she never said so.

"Whatever you want to do is precisely what's best for the baby," she told me. "Any tension you feel won't be good for her . . . or him." She desperately wanted a granddaughter. After four sons and two grandsons, she was ready for pink and ribbons and afternoons baking with a little girl on a stool beside her.

She told me, "I nursed for a few days. I didn't like it, so I stopped. Nobody breastfed back then, and you guys turned out okay."

Laney would swipe her palms together dismissively—washing her hands of the question. She wanted to discuss crib linens or how often she could come and be with me while I was on maternity leave. She let me know in no uncertain terms that her beloved oldest son was being a bully on the subject of breastfeeding, and that I should ignore him. She even rallied her friends to call me with their breastfeeding-wasn't-for-me-either stories.

Somehow my expectant state came to the attention of the La Leche League chapter near my home. I assumed my employer, big on preventive health care and with a comprehensive maternity program, had sent them my name.

The introductory call came to the house. My first mistake was not thanking them for their courtesy and hanging up.

"Do you have any concerns about feeding your baby?" the woman asked.

"No," I said.

"We'd love for you to drop by for coaching," she offered. "When are you due?"

I told her.

"Typically, we get together before the baby arrives, and then, of course, if you have any problems, we can stop by."

Figuring the truth (or something close to it) was best, I told her I was considering not breastfeeding.

"Oh, but you're missing a real opportunity if you only pump," she said, trying to sound upbeat.

I inhaled deeply, my hand clammy where it held the phone.

"I'm pretty sure I'll be using formula," I said, and waited.

"As a supplement?" she asked, her voice tensing.

"Only formula," I said.

There was silence, and then disbelief.

"No-no-no-no-no-no-no-no," she wailed. "But you *have* to."

I held the phone away from my ear. Mitch looked at me questioningly.

It's for you, I felt the urge to tell him, and then wondered if he'd been the one to pass them my name.

My personal decision became the cause célèbre of the League, or so it seemed. The calls didn't stop. At least their intrusion was more or less sanctioned. I could have cut them off, and I didn't. But then there were the people on the street, or on the elevator, or at the company Christmas party, people I'd never seen before, inquiring—as though for directions—whether I was planning to nurse. The people with the temerity to smooth their hands over my belly *while* they asked my breastfeeding plans made me want to scream.

Mitch cheered them on silently.

And it would be a nice story if I said I was transformed the moment my oldest was born and they put her on top of me, wrapped in pilly hospital flannel, her head covered by a cotton watch cap. The truth is, I was transformed. *Giddy* is the word that comes to mind. Her ears alone were miracles, petal-shaped and thin as paper.

If there was a moment I might have succumbed to Mitch's wishes and gotten over my inhibitions, it was then.

"At least give it a chance," he said, waving my bundled baby girl in front of my bosom, joking, I suppose, but also hoping she might latch on magnetically and something in me, some untapped urge, would take over. But by then the matter was settled in my mind for eternity. Mitch resigned himself soon enough. I couldn't fault him for his wish. At least we weren't fighting anymore.

And there was something satisfying about our both being able to feed the girls when they were infants. I loved watching Mitch with each of our daughters in turn, filling the crook of his arm as he fed her, and then the two of them lying on the couch, baby on Daddy's belly, snoozing peacefully.

This team parenting is still our style today: complementary, checking and balancing, picking up where the other leaves off. I am certain Mitch would have nursed our babies himself, if only he'd had the right parts.

Now, I wonder how I was able to hold my ground. And I confess I am wistful that I didn't give breastfeeding a whirl. No big regret, but an awareness of a missed opportunity. If, by some miracle of nature, I were to get pregnant today, I might even give breastfeeding a try.

I would breastfeed because it's a good thing to do. I would like to think, even if those heebie-jeebies struck again, that I would shake them off and be a little brave. I am mystified that more women haven't opted out, that so many are able to push through any misgivings or discomfort they have. I know I can't be alone in my feelings—although I might have felt alone on some late nights years ago.

As for my girls, they are incredible. Each one is tall and blond and has a mind as sharp as a tack. Among their loves are dogs and snakes, soccer and rowing, musicals and mathematics. Health issues? There have been a few. One had a bad bout of pneumonia in the third grade; another, enough ear infections that I felt compelled to have her hearing tested (the results were normal). I've taken the kids to the doctor no more than most other mothers I know—breastfeeders virtually all.

If I do have a regret, it's that my daughters won't have me as a positive role model when it is their turn to think about feeding their babies. (And if, after weighing their options, they choose not to nurse, I don't want to hear one word that might cause them stress.)

Do I think they should breastfeed my grandchildren? Yes, I do. I would like them to try, at least. And if they try it, I would like someone they love and trust and can count on unconditionally to stand next to them and say, "Let me help." And I'd like that person to be me. I won't know much from personal experience, but maybe we'll be able to figure it out together.

✳

Patricia Berry is a writer, columnist, and editor whose features and columns have appeared in *The New York Times, Working Mother, New Jersey Life, This Old House Magazine, ADDitude,* and other publications. A founding editor of *Sports Illustrated for Kids,* she is now at work on her first novel. She lives in New Jersey with her husband and three daughters.

CALLING IT QUITS

Pamela Kruger

When I think about breastfeeding my daughter, one scene immediately comes to mind: me, sitting on our living room couch, braless, shirtless, with my newborn baby positioned just so on a pillow in my lap. This is where I am sitting when my husband leaves for work in the morning and when he arrives home at night.

"Have you moved at all from that spot today?" my husband teases, when he comes home.

I promptly leap up and hand over our baby, who proceeds to whimper, then wail, until she is walked endlessly around our apartment or is back at my breast. While I don't laugh at his joke, I am comforted by it. I know that if he shared some of my crazy fears—that forever on, my days and nights would consist of no sleep, no work, no conversation, only nursing—he would not be trying to make me laugh. He would be consulting doctors, taking us to the hospital, maybe even calling 911. The fact that my husband is able to find humor in the situation says to me that he believes there will be a happy conclusion—although at the moment, I can't imagine how.

*   *

When I was pregnant, I devoured books and articles about motherhood. I was terrified by much of what I read—diapers, fifth disease, sleep deprivation, abusive nannies. But nursing was not on my list of worries. That was supposed to be easy, natural, something mothers have been doing for centuries until corporate interests duped us into paying for what our bodies can create for free. I knew that nursing was supposed to make kids happier, healthier, smarter. I'd read the gooey testimonials from women about the magical relationships they had developed with their babies because of breastfeeding. I was sure that I would be one of them.

That breastfeeding "on demand" would make getting a good night's sleep impossible, prevent me from working, and all but eliminate my husband's role in caregiving didn't occur to me.

I hadn't seen the studies showing that more than two-thirds of working mothers quit nursing after they go back to work, and that many women who continue nursing are out of the work force completely. I hadn't yet wondered why breastfeeding—and related attachment philosophies, which suggest that babies can be physically and emotionally scarred by separation from their mothers—had become de rigueur at precisely the same time that large numbers of mothers were employed outside the home. Those realizations do not come until later, after much anguish, anxiety, guilt, and self-doubt, when my milk has long since stopped flowing.

*   *

Soon after coming home from the hospital, I figure out that Emily is not latching on and is losing weight. I am frantic with worry. Someone suggests that I hire a lactation consultant. I hire several, spending hours and hundreds of dollars with these women to learn how to nourish my child. Normally, I am almost pathologically modest, but sheer exhaustion and abject terror have reduced me to an almost primal state. Topless, and without a trace of self-consciousness, I allow one stranger after another to poke and squeeze my areola as casually as if they were touching my knees.

Soon, Emily learns to latch on. I am relieved that she is gaining weight, but nursing on demand is draining me. While my mother and her peers were advised to put their babies on napping and feeding schedules (and leave their children in playpens while they went about their lives), the experts I consult preach the virtues of adapting to a baby's rhythms. Feeding on demand will stimulate milk production, the baby books and lactation consultants tell me. Echoing the precepts of attachment parenting, they recommend keeping my baby close to me at all times so that she will feel secure and connected. Co-sleeping, I am told, is a good idea, and when my baby is awake I should keep her in a baby carrier strapped to my body.

I comply for a while. The problem is, Emily demands to be fed around the clock. She isn't colicky but a "grazer." Emily snacks and then dozes off at my breast. If I put her down, she screeches. I try to follow her schedule and take short "power" naps. I go about my day "wearing" my daughter in the baby carrier. All of it is making me crazy and ready to snap.

I am weepy. I cannot think or talk about anything but Emily's nursing. Spending every minute of the day attached at

the hip to my baby is making me doubt my instincts and judgment, lose sense of who I am. I will not leave our apartment
without Emily for even a few minutes for fear that she might
become hungry. I talk endlessly about the difficulties of nursing and in embarrassing detail—how sore my areola is, how my
nipples are cracking—to my husband, editor, friends, sister,
neighbors, and really almost any other woman I know who will
listen. My husband, seeing his wife drift away, lost in a miasma
of fears and tears, puts his foot down, or at least tries to.

"Give her a pacifier," he says. "Let me give her a bottle."

I refuse, reciting chapter and verse what I've learned about
the risks of "nipple confusion" (namely: Since it is easier to get
milk through an artificially made nipple, some babies, when
bottle-fed, may forget how to nurse—or become "confused"—
and come to prefer the bottles to the real thing).

Every once in a while—I think it is during my weak moments, but perhaps it is my survival instinct surfacing—I consult the pediatrician and lactation consultants and my baby
books, looking for permission to quit.

Will it be okay if I stop after three weeks, four, six, nine
weeks? I ask. How long do I really need to do this?

No one tells me that I won't be harming my child by bottle
feeding. In fact, they seem to suggest the contrary, by reiterat-
ing (as if I needed reminding) the long list of supposed health
benefits of nursing to babies: strengthened immune system,
higher IQ, even reduced risk of sudden infant death syndrome.
(It is only years later that I learn that some of these "benefits"
are based on shaky science, but I will explain this later.)

My doctor recommends that I breastfeed for the first year,
but with much badgering I finally drag out of him that "perhaps" the most significant health advantages occur during the

first three months of nursing. (Studies showed that the post-partum milk, called colostrum, provides the baby with anti-bodies against common respiratory and intestinal infections, and that women who have breastfed for even three months are less likely to develop premenopausal breast cancer.)

I am holding on to that three-month number, but the lac-tation consultants, La Leche League volunteers, and baby books I consult are relentless advocates, so confident are they of the superiority of nursing. Behind their backs I call them "nursing Nazis," though they are always kind and understanding. They want to help me succeed. They want me to believe that I can succeed. Yes, it is inconvenient and frustrating to have to run back home in the middle of a grocery run or your first coffee with a friend because your baby suddenly starts wailing for your breast. They tell me about women who suffered as I did early on but grew to love nursing and breastfed through the toddler years. Even determined adoptive mothers manage to induce a milk supply; the system they use—involving tubes connected to the breast—seems to me to be bordering on masochistic, but what do I know?

Persevere, my nursing guides say, *it will get easier.*

I persevere. Through two cases of mastitis. Plugged ducts. Milk blisters. All kinds of misery. Don't get me wrong: There are moments when nursing brings me pure pleasure. With my daughter nuzzled to my breast, gazing into my eyes, I experi-ence moments of euphoria, bliss even. I am amazed and proud at what my body can do for my child.

Such moments are few and fleeting, though, overshadowed by the dark gloom settling over me, as I see no way back to work or my old self. Steeped as I am in the literature of the nursing mamas, I know that pumping is looked down upon, just barely a notch above formula feeding, lacking the bonding and nurturing that come only when the baby is at the mother's breast.

But as much as I hate to admit it, I do not want to be the only one getting up in the middle of the night to feed my daughter. One day, when Emily is perhaps four weeks old, I buy a $250 pump and hook myself up to it.

"Oh God, that looks medieval," my husband says.

"If men could nurse, we'd have a better contraption than this, wouldn't we?" I grumble, as I pump away.

An hour later, I hand over a bottle to my husband and leave for a walk around the neighborhood. I feel as though I'm missing an appendage and rush back home. But I continue to pump. My husband feeds Emily here and there. So do a babysitter, my siblings, and our parents. The heres and theres become more frequent, and, sure enough, by the time Emily is three months old, she develops "nipple confusion."

Or perhaps she isn't confused at all. Maybe she knows exactly what she wants.

Dirty secret: So do I.

I quit pumping altogether when Emily is four months old, one month better, I comfort myself, than the doctor ordered.

*　*

Bottle feeding allows me to return to work. It enables me to get a decent night's sleep and share caregiving more equally with my husband. Still, for months after quitting, I feel guilty and ashamed. Nursing was my first test as a mother, and I'd failed at it.

It wasn't until I began sharing my feelings that I realized I wasn't alone. One woman I know tells me that nursing was so painful that she cried every time she breastfed her son. Another nursed for six weeks, and then quit and promptly went into a depression. "I was convinced I was a bad mother," she says.

Years later, I've come to realize that, for me and many other women I know, nursing was just the beginning of that pointless and punishing quest to become the Perfect Mother. Pressure, judgment, and worry form a constant backdrop for mothers today. One day a study tells us we shouldn't leave our kids in daycare for more than twenty hours a week, or they'll become aggressive and unruly. Another day we hear that children whose parents aren't involved with their homework are more likely to be academic failures.

When we adopt our daughter, Annie, five years after Emily's birth, I feel relieved that I am not expected to nurse, but still I find myself fending off the barrage of "shoulds," the sense that somehow I should be doing more or something different as a parent.

We live in a culture saturated in mother-blame; virtually every decision we make as mothers is scrutinized, usually in un forgiving ways. Perhaps this has always been the case (mothers in the 1950s were blamed for autism, homosexuality, and a host of other "ills"). But the expectations for mothers seem to have been ratcheted up several notches, as more of us are working outside the home. A good mother today doesn't simply give her child age-appropriate toys—she has "floor time." She also purées organic vegetables for her baby, nurses until her baby is at least one year old, makes Halloween costumes from scratch, and certainly doesn't "outsource" child care. I've drawn the line at feeding my kids at McDonald's, and I try to buy only organic foods, but my daughters have had their share of chicken fingers and pizza dinners, have been in daycare or with a babysitter from infancy pretty much through kindergarten, and have been sent to watch a Disney DVD more times than I care to count because I couldn't bear to play Barbies with them.

Probably most of us fall short in one way or another, but unfortunately we internalize the ideals and are quick to wag our fingers at each other. I remember reading an essay in a parenting magazine in which a mother confessed she didn't nurse; readers later attacked her for being uninformed and selfish. The medical establishment can be just as harsh. Not too long ago a national public-health campaign compared a woman's failure to nurse to smoking during pregnancy—and worse. "You'd never take risks before your baby is born. Why start after?" the announcer intoned, after showing a pregnant woman riding and falling off a mechanical bull during ladies' night at a bar.

While some in the national media criticized the tenor of the campaign, I didn't see any question the underlying assumption that nursing brings better health. Yet many scientists vigorously dispute that idea. As an August 2007 article in the *Journal of Health Politics, Policy and Law* put it, the research is "inconsistent, lacks strong associations, and does not account for plausible confounding variables, such as the role of parental behavior, in various health outcomes."

The notion that formula-fed babies have lower IQs, for instance, is based on studies that have been debunked in two major scientific reviews; the studies that purported to show a link between IQ and nursing failed to "satisfy basic methodological standards" and didn't consider other factors, such as whether mothers who nurse their babies may promote academic success in other ways. Virtually all of the health claims—that breastfeeding reduces the rates of respiratory illnesses, sudden infant death syndrome, and Type 2 diabetes—

have been under attack, either because of confounding variables or because better studies have refuted the conclusions altogether.

Reading this research, I've come to believe that the nursing-versus-formula debate is a lot like the paid-child-care-versus-parental-care debate and many of the other controversies swirling around child rearing: There is a lot of self-righteous moralizing about what children supposedly need, but in the end all we know for sure is that there isn't one superior way to mother. As clichéd and morally bankrupt as it may sound to some, I really believe we all need to make choices that work best for our families—for both parents and child.

So, if you are among those who have found nursing to be wonderful, good for you. Do I still wish it had been the easy and blissful experience I'd read about? You bet, but for whatever reason, it was not. I hope you will not judge me. Most important, I've learned to try, at least, not to judge myself.

✳

Pamela Kruger is a freelance writer, editor, and blogger whose work has been published in *The New York Times*, *Child*, *Parenting*, *Fast Company*, *The Huffington Post*, and several anthologies, including *A Love Like No Other: Stories from Adoptive Parents*, which she coedited with Jill Smolowe. She lives with her husband and their two daughters in New Jersey.

DRAINED

Jessica Restaino

Postpartum depression feels like you've swallowed a rusty anchor. It sits in your guts and colors everything—even the good stuff—with an awful rot. You're stuck and sometimes it's hard to breathe. But even with all its influence, the sadness isn't so obvious or easy to identify. My own journey through postpartum depression began murkily, an echo of what I saw as my first failures as a mother: birth and breastfeeding.

The events of Abby's birth were terrifying for me: a long, overdue labor, hours of pushing, and finally a gas mask over my face. Abby was born by rushed c-section while I was unconscious. My earliest memory is our first feeding the next morning. Still foggy and slow, I had no real sense that the process worked, but Abby seemed satisfied. Our few days in the hospital proceeded in similar obscurity. I never thought much about what was going on. The night nurse would tell me I needed my rest. I slept. A nurse woke me up each morning, and I'd put my baby to my breast. I fed Abby throughout the daytime hours and would part with her again at night. She gained an ounce, and I got my sleep.

Today I realize the depression started before I left the hospital. But I had heard that sometimes women feel ambivalent about their new babies in the first days. So when I noticed that my husband, Ryan, seemed so in love with our daughter, I wondered why he loved her so much, but I was not ready to admit that I didn't feel the same way. Perhaps I didn't immediately feel the waves of love—that intense maternal connection—because of the bruises under my eyes, my unsteady legs, my puffy skin. As we left the hospital, I wasn't yet frightened by my emotional blankness. I figured I just needed to heal physically and feel a bit more like myself.

But at home things got worse. Abby and I discovered that I had no milk for her at night. Confused and desperate, I tried nursing her nearly every hour while she screamed hungrily. I remember staring down at her—2:00 A.M., 3:00 A.M., 4:00 A.M.— bewildered by her crying. I sobbed along with her. After endless struggle, the outcome was a tidal wave of milk. By the end of the first week home, my breasts had clogged with hard knots, hot lumps I could feel like marbles beneath my blotchy red skin. I read furiously, trying to find a solution: a hot shower, a heating pad, massaging the lumps while she nursed. I started running a fever. My breasts became so hard and swollen that Abby struggled to draw milk from them. In my mind I allowed myself to admit, silently, *I hate this. I hate nursing.* I longed to utter the words aloud but couldn't bear to hear myself.

During that first week home, I started to get scared. It wasn't just the breastfeeding that—already—wasn't working. The love on Ryan's face in the hospital—that staggering, forever love—wasn't in me. I still hadn't fallen in love with my daughter. I started to worry out loud, "What if I can't love her enough?" Ryan assured me I already did. Why didn't I feel it?

How could he know? What was wrong with me? Fear of not loving Abby settled into my core. I hadn't thought this could happen. But I also hadn't imagined that I'd be unconscious for her birth, or that breastfeeding would seem impossible. In those first days home, my one assurance in the world happened each time Ryan handed me our baby to nurse. He loved her enough, sure, but he couldn't feed her. When she cried he'd look to me. Though painfully aware that something wasn't right, I was her source of nourishment, and she seemed to know it.

And so I kept trying, despite the fact that I knew my body had not taken to nursing. I longed to make nursing work and to feel better, so I made an appointment with my doctor. She quickly proclaimed that I had an infection and prescribed antibiotics. I did three rounds, and each time I'd feel better for two days, and then a new clog would form, spiking my fever again. Abby would cry and arch as her nursing efforts were not easily rewarded. Overwhelmed and perhaps badly advised, I pumped milk endlessly and put it into bottles for her. Pumping provided immediate relief from the pain I couldn't stand anymore. But it also increased my milk production, causing my breasts to become even more engorged. In the mornings I'd awake to peel off my soaked shirt. I found myself stuck in a maddening cycle. Eight weeks later I quit nursing completely, with a freezer full of milk, little bags lined up like casualties of war.

As my milk dried up, the physical pain lifted. In the quiet that followed, I knew I was somehow still sick. I quickly realized the pain was deep, a scary sadness in my throat, my stomach. This sadness was a kind of physical ache, too, but one haunted and fanned by my thoughts. I certainly wasn't a "natural" mother, and maybe, if I was meant to be a good mother, things like labor and delivery, like breastfeeding, would have come more easily to me. While I knew I'd make mistakes as a parent, throughout my pregnancy I took real comfort in the fact that my body seemed to know what it was doing. From the day my daughter was born, I started to believe this instinct didn't exist in me. Memories of her delivery and the infant formula stacked on top of my refrigerator screamed a simple message: I wasn't built for this. My mind raced with worry. What had I done to this helpless baby?

Terrified, I began to see all around me other women who seemed more naturally inclined to motherhood. Breastfeeding worked for everyone who tried, I was certain. I must not have tried hard enough. Other mothers pushed out their babies, if their bodies were built correctly. How could I have been unconscious? Why did I let that happen? All mothers fell in love, instantly, with their newborns. Everything was fine for everyone else. They all adjusted. They were so happy, so joyful. Things made sense. There was something wrong with me. While I tried to hide my inadequacy, I also believed in it, was certain of it.

I was preoccupied most of the time, fantasizing about what it would feel like to be a good mother. Even as I played with my healthy baby, I was far away. Friends had babies and nursed successfully, again and again. I was sure it was so easy for them. At their good news, I was immediately lost in myself. I felt as if I were underwater, hearing only muffled sounds and unable to breathe. I couldn't move naturally. I couldn't shut off my brain. I was selfishly deep in my own mind, and I didn't know how to get out of it. I knew Abby was doing well, and this made me vividly aware of my own disproportionate sadness. How could I not appreciate the growing, beautiful child I had? When I posed this question to myself, my answer immediately—irrationally—would be that if I had been able to make breastfeeding work, I wouldn't feel this way. The sadness, I thought, was my punishment for my first failures at motherhood. While I was able to care for my baby, I was unable to forgive myself. My feelings, so terrifyingly real, were distorted and overblown.

I can say this now, nearly three years later. But I didn't have this kind of conviction then. Inside I felt only the heat of a guilty secret, a knowing sense that somehow I had cheated my baby. My mind swirled with blame: I had taken the easy way out. I handed over all control to the doctors when she was born. I wasn't there for her. I let her arrive in the world alone. I didn't stick with nursing long enough. I gave in to physical pain, when I could have just soldiered through. The infection would have gone away eventually. If only I could take back the quitting, could fix it, could start over with breastfeeding, I was sure that the deepest hurt, the scary knowledge that I wasn't built for motherhood, would be undone. But I couldn't go back. I had stopped making milk and was empty. Whenever I got lost in these thoughts, a sharp knife rose up from my guts and into my mouth, choking me. At the time I was terrified by my emotions and desperate to make them go away, to feel the joy of a new baby. My sadness became a source of guilt.

My worries from the first week of motherhood, that I wouldn't love Abby enough, soon grew into an unwieldy obsession with her well-being. My love was fear. And I was so scared about anything bad happening to Abby that I knew I finally loved her intensely. I bolted up in bed at night, tortured by mental images of my baby getting hurt. Always, in my mind's scenarios, I was just missing her as she fell from the couch or off the changing table. I could feel the air through my fingers, the missing weight of her body. Wide awake, I'd stand by her crib and watch her sleep, desperate for the reassurance that she was unharmed. But I couldn't shake the fear. Descending steps, I could feel Abby slipping out of my arms, my muscles loose and unreliable. This wasn't simply a fear of making mistakes as a new mother. I felt powerless that I couldn't protect Abby from unseen threats. I decided that mother love—this kind of love I had for my child—had broken me. I had lost the ability to play, to be hopeful, to be silly. I mourned these parts of myself quietly.

Abby's first year rolled on, despite my own struggles, because she was clearly a force of life meant to grow and be in the world. Before long I was thinking about her first birthday and yet still living with aching regret about giving up nursing and constant nervousness about Abby's safety. At Barnes & Noble I would go right to the motherhood magazines and flip pages until I could find an article about the benefits of breastfeeding. Immediately I was underwater again, hearing only my insides—my heart pounding, my own guilty self-awareness. I read these articles as proof that my daughter would surely get sick and that it would be my fault. I actually looked for them, almost to confirm my fears and punish myself. I fed my anxiety and my guilt endlessly and began to worry that I could never stop. Noisy questions tortured my thoughts: *Will I exist like this for the rest of my life? What happens when Abby is old enough to sense my sadness? What if she already can?*

A photo from that time still haunts me. It's really a picture of Abby, approaching the camera playfully, with her dad's baseball hat on her head. She's almost a year old in the picture, and obviously deliriously happy. In the background I sit on the floor, cross-legged. My posture is awful. But the worst of it is my face: drawn, tired, deeply sad. Sorrow had inscribed a heavy pain into my eyes, the bones of my face, my dry lips. No longer were there internal and external wounds. The lines of separation had simply blurred. I was one ache, physically, emotionally, and spiritually depressed. And while on some level I must have known this all year, the grainy image of myself, slumping behind my gleeful child, shocked me.

I sought help soon after and spent Abby's second year of life getting better. Therapy was hard, and because I had to schedule sessions while Abby was at daycare, I would go during the workday. I'd slip out for an hour and then return to teach a class, hoping students wouldn't notice that I looked as if I'd just been through an ugly breakup. In many ways that's what getting better was like. It was a breaking away from something deeply personal, deeply mine. The way the pain sifted out of me felt very slow. For a long time I was aware that the sadness was still there, in my gut, even when I felt a bit better. At times it flared up, even after a good stretch, agitated by reminders of breastfeeding—a friend's new baby nursing comfortably, a browse through the motherhood magazines, a news feature. In these moments I couldn't get the feelings of guilty hurt from my mind. Sometimes, in private, I caught myself actually shaking my head quickly from side to side, trying to physically expel the thoughts that I had come to hate.

I had a desperate drive to get better. My ongoing concern and regret over breastfeeding, in particular, angered and annoyed me. But this frustration wasn't enough to make it stop. Finally, my therapist gave me something to read about the connection that mothers with postpartum depression often have to breastfeeding. I saw myself. I remember that the author described the struggling mother's relationship to breastfeeding as the last lifeline, sometimes the only evidence, in the mother's distorted perception, of her worth to her child. Before I stopped breastfeeding, I already feared I was depressed. When I ended the breastfeeding relationship, I altogether unraveled.

I think some of that unraveling had deep roots in a maternal, biological drive that exceeds my own comprehension. But popular media's often careless messages about breastfeeding were damaging, too. In countless parenting magazines I saw sweeping claims about intelligence, about the prevention of diseases such as cancer and diabetes. These pieces are rarely tempered by honest disclaimers about the difficulties of doing convincing research on breastfeeding. Breast milk has lifesaving power in the developing world, where clean drinking water is scarce. But popular magazines, marketed to suburban mothers in the West, tend to overlook this staggering fact in exchange for weaker claims about the upper-middle-class child's seat in the gifted classroom. I think this sells breastfeeding short and is needlessly dangerous for mothers with postpartum depression.

As I healed, I slowly started to escape the grasp of such media, and my love changed again. Fear melted into joy and silliness. I still sit on the edge of my seat as Abby chews a too-large bite of apple. But I have also found myself trusting her more. My nearly three-year-old, with her "big-girl" underwear and her love of questions, is growing into a person. She wants to figure things out for herself; she is curious and even daring. In the moments when I watch her fumble with a zipper or walk alone into the toddler crowd at a birthday party, I get to love her on her terms. I think this is what I've learned most profoundly during my journey. What I saw as my "failures" as a new mother were just that: all mine. I found their traces on my face, not my daughter's. She is the girl who was born healthy and who grew and grew on infant formula. When I started to get better, I could see our wonderful separateness. I could see that she wasn't hurting, that it had been me, all this time, and only me. She wasn't there for her own birth; the pain was mine, not hers. I was sad about how things went; she wasn't. As I peeled back the layers of my depression, I realized that it had been, always, a battle with my own expectations.

Ultimately, I learned more than simply to see myself in a more favorable light. I learned to look beyond myself—at my daughter and the way her lips curl when she gets a joke. At her eyes, those deep disks, when she's proud of herself. I now believe the best we can do for mothers—depressed or not—is to celebrate our distinctiveness. All over the world, mothers, and even their babies, are distinct from one another, and they do things in many different ways. And, in a way, this unifies us. This is the kind of thesis statement that, as an English professor, I see on student papers. In a huff, I scribble in the margin, "Can you get more specific?!" But let's leave it this time. We are, as mothers, that profound.

✳

Jessica Restaino is assistant professor of English at Montclair State University. Her scholarly work focuses on preparation of new teachers, writing pedagogy, and the political thought of Hannah Arendt. She is the proud mother of Abby.

IN THE LAND OF
MILK AND MONEY

Jill Hamburg Coplan

We do not accept the traditional assumption that a woman has to choose between marriage and motherhood, on the one hand, and serious participation in industry or the professions on the other. We question the present expectation that all normal women will retire from job or profession for 10 or 15 years, to devote their full time to raising children, only to reenter the job market at a relatively minor level.

> —Statement of Purpose, The National
> Organization for Women, adopted
> at its organizing conference,
> Washington, DC, October 29, 1966

I hold NOW's founding manifesto, a faded mimeograph, in my hand. It arrived recently in a carton of 1970s feminist papers from Aunt Geri, who is moving. Geri Raichel—a founding member of a New Jersey NOW chapter, head of public-school gifted programs, who wrote her doctoral dissertation on gender equality in elementary education. I appreciate this document. I was a 1970s child feminist, discovering "women's lib" in fourth grade. I collected Susan B. Anthony coins, and as a teen I pitched a tent at the Seneca Falls Women's Encampment for a Future of Peace and Justice. Of course I didn't *accept the traditional assumption that a woman has to choose . . . between motherhood . . . and the professions.* What idiot would?

Now I'm forty-two, sitting beside Geri's box, reading: *We question that all normal women will retire for 10 or 15 years to devote their full time to raising children.* My oldest child is nearly eight. And I am in my eighth year of child-raising semiretirement.

He was born on Thanksgiving, 1999, and a few weeks home from the hospital, with my hopes of going back to my job still intact, my accountant gave me the first hint there would be trouble in paradise. My spouse and I both made middle-class salaries, mine from editing a magazine and, before that, working as an entry-level newspaper and wire-service reporter. The hours were long, but I was extremely privileged— riding jeeps into war zones, skim-reading six newspapers a day, meeting Hillary Clinton at the White House, flying to Europe to interview ministers, taking sources or writers to lunch. Once a talk show had even invited me on to discuss a controversial story. My accountant explained that if I returned to work full time, child-care expenses and taxes would erase almost all my take-home pay. Of course, I could leave my baby from 7:00 to 7:00 if I wanted to, but there would be little to show for it at the end of the year but dry-cleaning bills and train fare.

Clue two that things might not pan out: I was making the rounds of work-related conferences and holiday events, baby in a sling. He traveled well—he could always be calmed by nursing—but while maternity office wear was easy to find, business-like nursing clothes were not (I was so swollen with milk that few shirts could get over those inflated boobs). So I went where there was privacy: cramped and not particularly clean toilet stalls. (And while I found that options were lacking in those office buildings, restaurants, and hotels, studies show that "workplace facilities and support" are far worse for pink-collar service and factory workers, who must choose straightaway whether to breastfeed or to work. At least I wasn't getting fired—not yet.)

The women's movement hadn't seen mothering this way. "There really is nothing," said NOW President Aileen C. Hernandez, in her 1971 keynote speech at the group's fifth annual convention, "that makes us uniquely able to rear children."

By chance I was a milk overproducer, which meant the baby wouldn't starve, but my ability had a downside: If I got preoccupied and missed a feeding, which was happening continually, on came mastitis, a breast infection that hits like a sudden flu with 104-degree fevers, aches, and dizziness. I got it four times in the first two months. Get it a fifth time, my OB said, and she'd check me into a hospital. An expensive lactation consultant (not covered by insurance) put it this way: If I wanted to breastfeed—and I did, for the baby's and my own physical and emotional well-being—then nursing and resting were about to become my full-time job, for the next two months, three months, maybe more.

Conventional wisdom says establishing regular milk flow takes six to eight weeks. But for some women calibrating Mom's supply to Baby's demand can take up to six months. This includes people who, while preparing to return to work, stockpile milk by pumping extra. The body can be easily fooled into making enough for two kids. Along with everything else I did wrong, I was guilty of that error, too.

But six months off? I'd envisioned a standard corporate six-week maternity leave, but it turned out my boobs had other plans. When my leave ended, I asked my boss if I could become a part-timer, and she said no. (Companies are generally too stupid to offer flextime and part-time work routinely—though study after study shows they lead to greater productivity and lower turnover and training costs, which result in measurably higher profits.) In the shock of being unemployed, I learned what other secrets my boobs had been keeping, like the feel-good hormone oxytocin, the natural opiate that floods the brain after orgasm and breastfeeding. Also that one could (in my case, with two kids who each breastfed for two years) nurse off one hundred pounds. That I'd significantly reduce my risk of breast cancer. That I had an infallible way to calm an often savage little beast. And that there would be extra emotional closeness between mother and baby, which, studies during the past decade say, is driven by breastfeeding hormones and is possibly also linked to the constant skin-on-skin contact necessitated by breastfeeding. (Research finds that nursing mothers also do more with their babies when they aren't nursing—more holding, rocking, speaking, sleeping.) Being apart for eleven hours, day after day, seemed incredibly painful. Is this what the founders of the women's movement intended?

So I breastfed exclusively for about six months, as medical orthodoxy says you should, and took up teaching, plus, often in the wee hours, writing and editing. I was a privileged, educated worker, fortunate that I could pay the bills working mostly from home, nights and weekends, with a few hours of babysitting, a spouse, and a grandmother to cover child care. I was lucky the publishing business (beaten down by the Internet and hobbled by layoffs) was freelancer friendly. To breastfeed, I'd become a casual, an adjunct, lining up gigs. While my babies thrived, my career went on life support.

We question the present expectation that all normal women will retire . . . only to reenter the job market at a relatively minor level, reads the manifesto I hold in my hand. In so many ways I owe the manifesto writers a debt of gratitude. But I've just got a middle-class nursing mother's blues: My Social Security and retirement contributions have plummeted, irreplaceably. My much-needed income has turned unreliable. And God knows what a career on-ramp might look like, exactly, after eight years in the wilderness.

When I say that 1970s feminists could not have foreseen these boob-related issues, I mean that overcoming breastfeeding problems wasn't part of their pursuit of full equality. First, prevailing medical advice at the time wasn't to nurse for the year or two now recommended by U.S. and international pediatric bodies. Though feminist health activists would change this in time, most of these women probably hadn't done it themselves.

Perhaps more powerful was the prevailing philosophy. Such pesky matters of nature were understood to be what had stood in women's way for so long. The less said about them, perhaps, the better. "We have been brainwashed and we have been structured and we have been carefully trained and formed over generations," Hernandez said in her 1971 keynote, "to be what they now say is an inherent part of our nature." *Nature*—it was almost a dirty word. Look past those breasts, our troublesome bodies, our sexual biology, our childbearing—and see us as equals. Women had had enough of being circumscribed by gross biological differences, by messy bodily functions. A new social determinism of nurture would trump retrograde old biological determinism. The genetic code hadn't been cracked yet. Who knew how much of each of us would turn out to be hardwired? People were seen as entirely malleable, sometimes with tragic results (consider the doctors who believed they could successfully reassign intersex babies, simply by choosing a sex for them and doing genital surgery early enough).

Breastfeeding was coded politically conservative, for the stay-at-home, right-wing woman. In mother's milk was the weight of traditionalism, natalism, the oppressive family model the movement wanted to do away with: Dad, breadwinner; Mom, homemaker. In its place the revolution would put curative androgyny: "It is our central task to liberate the positive aspects of the so-called 'masculine' in girls and women, and the so-called 'feminine' in boys and men, for individuals and institutions to be healthy and whole," declared NOW President Wilma Scott Heide in her 1974 national conference speech.

As much as the movement accomplished in education, in law, in combating violence against women, the demands of our nature were its blind spot. *We question the present expectation that all normal women will retire.* The president of the Center for Work-Life Policy, Sylvia Ann Hewlett, questioned it, too. She found that when "highly qualified women" take "extended" maternity leaves, only 40 percent ever make it back to full-time employment. (No one has checked whether these subjects breastfed, but older age and higher education and income suggest they would have.) Other new research shows that women who take time off lose, on average, more than $1 million in income over the course of their careers. There is something that makes us *uniquely able to rear children*, and it can make a difference, a humongous difference, during arguably the most productive decades of a woman's working life.

Scene: the august halls of the Council on Foreign Relations, an exclusive organization housed in an Upper East Side townhouse. My second baby is old enough that I've gotten away for a daylong conference and even managed to squeeze into appropriate attire. Now, leaking milk while impeccably groomed investment bankers, foundation types, and caterers skitter about, I'm trying to find an outlet where I can plug in the portable Pump In Style slung over my shoulder before I explode. I bump into George Soros. Condoleezza Rice takes the stage. There is no outlet available anywhere, so I leave.

Problems with pumping rise steeply as a working woman's economic power falls. A 2007 survey by the nonprofit National Women's Health Resource Center found that only 23 percent of women in retail and service jobs are nursing at six months, versus 42 percent of mothers higher on the economic ladder, and the reasons women who were surveyed gave all had to do with pumping: lack of privacy at work to pump, lack of refrigeration to store breast milk, inadequate number of breaks to pump, discomfort storing or cleaning pump supplies in front of coworkers, anxiety about discussing breastfeeding needs at work.

Exclusive breastfeeding for the first several months is now a national health-care priority, thanks to numerous benefits that are so well known they hardly bear repeating, yet public policies that would make it possible for more than a small minority to do it lag behind those in developing countries. And changing this is on almost no politician's agenda. (The exception is Sen. Christopher Dodd of Connecticut, who spearheaded passage of the landmark Family and Medical Leave Act, providing workers unpaid leave for new-baby care and other family needs. Shortly after announcing his 2008 presidential ambitions, Dodd cosponsored a bill to give caregivers six weeks of *paid* leave, with costs to be split among employers, workers, and the federal government. At this writing the bill is stalled in committee.)

Aunt Geri had her own personal work-life solution that allowed her to finish her PhD. When she had two babies in the late 1960s, her mother, Grandma Rose, came to look after the children. When Geri shipped me her archives forty years later, she was packing for a cross-country move that would bring her full circle: She was going to care for her grandchild, so her own daughter could complete her advanced medical training.

Few people have such wells of generosity to tap. Still, it's far from the scenario activists had in mind in the heady days of the 1970s women's movement, or the future I envisioned as a little girl, when I hoped to follow in the footsteps of Elizabeth Cady Stanton or Nellie Bly. Now, surrounded by nearly half-century-old pamphlets and ditto-sheet papers, the simple shape of those hopes is so clear that my inability to realize them feels as raw and jarring as if I had left my magazine yesterday, rather than a decade ago. Despite my privileges and my good fortune of working from home, I still haven't come to terms with having to leave the world where I thought I belonged. I sometimes imagine going back, and if I had to I would. Yet I don't regret the way I raised my babies. Knowing all I know about breast-feeding, in good conscience I couldn't have raised them differently. But I still can hardly believe things turned out this way.

※

Jill Hamburg Coplan formerly worked as a wire-service and newspaper reporter in the Middle East and Africa and wrote the "Work & Family" column for BusinessWeek.com. Now she edits for *BusinessWeek*, teaches journalism at New York University, writes for magazines, works on a novel, and runs after her five- and eight-year-old sons.

LIFTED

Stephanie Kilroy

My infant daughter, Zoey-Cate, is seven days old and she has spent most of her life crying. "I know why she's crying," my four-year-old daughter, Leilani, tells me, peering into the baby's gaping mouth as she screams. "She's sad because she doesn't have any teeth."

This may well be the case, but I am also concerned that something else is wrong with my baby.

Since returning home from the hospital, life has changed for our family. My husband, Brian, and I have been replaying an exhausting performance, the feature role in this drama played by Zoey. She has no lines to memorize; she cries in act one, nurses enter in act two. Brian's and my roles remain fixed. We play it straight—the unassuming parents under siege—rendered helpless by an angry, screaming baby. Our daughter's arrival on the scene hasn't quite been the welcome-home love fest we had imagined.

*　　*

"She's been crying for twenty minutes," Brian tells me, his jaw tight, holding the baby stiffly in his arms. Twenty minutes is the amount of time the pediatrician has given us, as a guideline, to allow the baby to cry before tending to her. Crying isn't quite the appropriate term for what Zoey is doing at the moment; her extreme agitation might qualify her as a good candidate for an exorcism. Brian delivers her to me as one might hand over a dirty dish that needs cleaning. "She must need The Boob." I play the role of The Boob, a mobile, twenty-four-hour diner with breast milk on tap, ready to serve the nursing-on-demand needs of my daughter.

"But I just fed her," I reply, defensively. I don't need another dirty dish to clean. My breasts are far from engorged; they are soft, like two overripe nectarines. I refer to my nursing journal. The baby has just sucked from each breast for twenty minutes, through back-to-back episodes of annoyingly overgroomed preschoolers singing on the *Barney and Friends* show. Leilani stands an arm's length from the television, entranced, swaying gently to the music. She has a fear of people dressed as mascots, but strangely she loves Barney and his shiny white teeth.

The shrieks rev up and take on a high-rpm pitch, like a vacuum cleaner with a sock trapped in its mouth. "Honey," Brian says, raising his voice above the din. I turn to examine the source of the crying, our baby beloved. Zoey is a perfect shade of eggplant, a pinched and rigid screaming thing. She is our household's very own anti-Barney: purple, but certainly not nice, without a single note of anything singsong sweet coming out of her mouth. She is a menacing presence, this beautiful baby; she threatens and torments. The cry-screaming persists; I unhook my nursing bra and fold Zoey's face in towards my breast, and she latches on immediately, grunting hungrily as she nurses. My nipple aches from her tremendous pull.

This is the drama Brian and I have been playing out in our household, matinee and evening performances both: frantic crying followed by hungry nursing. Brian peeks in to confirm that the baby is breastfeeding, then steps away, the haunted look in his eyes dissolving a bit, but not entirely. He is still worried, anticipating more crying. There will always be a next time. It's not a matter of *if*, but *when*.

* *

When the baby is ten days old, a nurse pays us a routine visit from the hospital to give her a follow-up examination. For ten days I have lived, with hairy armpits and perineal pain, on our tweedy green couch, nursing Zoey. Both flaps of my nursing bra are open, and my bare breasts poke out the open holes, like two yoked oxen. My nipples feel like raw burn wounds beneath the fabric of my flannel pajamas.

Brian and Leilani pass by, trailing a backpack and lunch box, and pepper me with kisses on their way out the door. Brian has temporarily taken over driving the carpool. My once-full life has narrowed in focus and is now centered on breastfeeding. I pay bills and read books, all while sitting on the couch, my baby ball and chain either screaming or hanging from my breast, nursing.

And the *stuff*: the abandoned Boppy pillow, a stack of fresh burp cloths, half-read magazines, and protein bars in a weedy sprawl around my feet. I have established a nursing base camp, and I have hunkered down to acclimate to my new environment. I am isolated from the world around me, as if on a barren, rocky ledge scattered with empty oxygen bottles at seventeen thousand feet.

*   *

The nurse, Brenda, arrives promptly at 9:30. Her glossy brown hair is tied back in a neat ponytail. Clearly a woman who is getting plenty of sleep, she smiles radiantly. In my exhaustion I have forgotten the subject of her visit—the baby—and I believe she is my Fairy Lactation Consultant, come to wave her magic wand and save me from my misery.

"How's the nursing?" she asks, conversationally, unloading the portable scale from its case.

"It's going," I venture, doing my best to imitate good cheer, but I stop short, suddenly afraid I might cry. I tell Brenda that I'm having trouble. My nipples are cracked and bleeding. I ask if she wants to see them.

"Oh, that's not necessary," Brenda tells me, as if waving off dessert after a rich meal. "But there might be a problem with her latching on."

I am experienced enough at breastfeeding to know a good latch from a bad one. My problem extends beyond latching on. I think of the dairy industry's famed advertisement: GOT MILK? I'm not sure that I do. After marathon sessions with the breast pump, I'm hard-pressed to deliver more than a thin film of milk into the pump's receptacle. And when Zoey nurses, it's as if she's sucking on the side of an inflated balloon. All her energy is spent, and she's getting something, but I don't think it's enough.

I tell Brenda that, two years ago, after weaning Leilani, I had had breast-lift surgery. I'm afraid my milk production has been compromised.

"You should probably talk to a lactation consultant," Brenda answers, carefully unswaddling Zoey. "Implants?"

I answer no. No implants, no reduction, just a lift.

Brenda looks at me thoughtfully. "If your nipples have not been removed and repositioned, you shouldn't have a problem."

You shouldn't have a problem. And yet I do. I have this baby, this disruptive, squalling complainer. She must be complaining for a reason.

I have talked to a couple of lactation consultants, both before and after having Zoey. They were both informed and supportive, and they told me that since my breast tissue was not removed, and my nipples were left intact, I could be successful at breastfeeding. A breast lift should not impinge on a mother's ability to feed her baby. *And keep at it,* they told me. *The more you feed, the better your supply.*

And I want to breastfeed. I want it to be the magical, meaningful experience it was for me when I nursed Leilani. But there is no magic here.

* *

I am no stranger to chafed nipples, to the rigorous demands of breastfeeding. I know that cracks, scabs, and bloody milk can all be a part of the break-in experience of nursing. When I first began breastfeeding, I felt as if my internal organs were being sucked out of me through my nipples. At times my nipple tissue had the mashed, grainy texture of ground beef. But, as many mothers do, I worked through it; soon my breasts toughened up to the point that I could probably have nursed a lion cub without flinching.

I breastfed Leilani exclusively for one year and weaned her

as she approached her second birthday. Her lips never touched a bottle, she never drank a drop of formula, and I credit her good health to every ounce of breast milk she swallowed. Her growth chart was an immaculate curve, a line connecting points over time in a perfect fiftieth-percentile arc. She never had an ear infection, rarely had a cold. I was sure these were all benefits lavished on her by my breast milk.

Breastfeeding had come so easily to me that I saw no reason why anyone else couldn't do it. So, very quickly I became a hard-core, "Breast Is Best"–bumper-sticker-wielding kind of mama, evangelizing the breast-milk gospel to anyone who would listen.

The flip side of my passion for breastfeeding was that I felt a bit superior. All those formula sinners out there needed to be *saved*, and perhaps it was my calling to spread the good news and to breastfeed proudly, and publicly, maybe converting along the way a few who had strayed from the path that nature had intended. I couldn't help but deliver a judgmental glance when a mom at a play date carefully ladled scoopfuls of formula into a bottle.

* *

After weaning Leilani, my breasts returned to their former size C, yet I had a textbook case of ptosis, commonly known as droop. Examining my breasts in the mirror, I began to draw certain parallels between my breasts and those of topless aboriginal women sometimes seen tending to open fires on National Geographic programs.

I toyed with the idea of getting a breast lift. The tipping point may have come after sharing what should have been an inconsequential morning shower with Leilani. "Mommy," she told me, poking my nipple as I bent over to shampoo her hair. "Mommy, your boobies are so long!" I recoiled. Her use of the words *boobies* and *long* in the same sentence seemed a frightening juxtaposition of two incongruous terms.

My breasts had sagged slightly since adolescence; breast-feeding Leilani only helped finalize their ruin. I blame it on genetics: Look up a few leafy branches of my family tree, and you'll find it ripe with grandmothers and great-aunts who suffered as well. Mine is a tribe with low-slung breasts. My expectations weren't unrealistic—I wasn't looking to morph into Pamela Anderson or get a night job at Hooters—I just wanted my breasts restored.

I didn't consider getting a breast lift a reckless act; I didn't think I would have any more children. I was thirty-one years old and a single mother, and Leilani was my only child. I approached my future with shrewd realism. The odds of getting married and having more children were slim. Hadn't studies been done? Didn't I stand a better chance of being struck by lightning than I did of finding a husband? So why wait on breast-lift surgery if I might never breastfeed again?

I had no way of knowing that in one year's time I would meet Brian, eventually get married, and have three more children in quick succession.

* *

I spent time in the library, flipping through pictures of gory medical procedures in order to learn more about mine. I was not able to find much in the literature that related specifically to breastfeeding after mastopexy, but what I did read indicated that I could successfully nurse after the procedure. I consulted with three different plastic surgeons before having my procedure. Out came the colorful diagrams; great care went into explaining the operation. *During the mastopexy procedure, the nipple will remain attached to the breast tissue at all times, in effect preserving the function of the breast and nipple.*

Each plastic surgeon I met with confirmed that I was a good candidate for a breast lift. As I sat naked from the waist up on an examination table, I was told that I had deflated, or "empty," breasts—that my breasts had excess skin in relation to their volume. My mind conjured up an image of a pair of tube socks, their toes filled with sand.

Then it came time to address my concerns about my ability to breastfeed after undergoing the lift procedure.

As a single mother who hadn't had a date in over two years, it seemed ludicrous to broach the topic, but there I was, explaining to a strange man in a white coat that although I had no husband or suitable prospects, there existed this remote possibility that I might . . . might . . . find a man—it was hard to suppress my own guffaws as I explained this to the doctor—and have more children, but I could hardly see it happening, as I spent most of my free time blowing bubbles on a parachute at Gymboree, or cleaning out the highchair.

The doctor stared blankly, looking for the tie-in, the wrap-up.

"I'm getting old," I told him. "I don't know any single men. But if I did find someone, and have children with him, I would like to breastfeed again."

Each doctor I consulted told me that I should be able to nurse a child after mastopexy. *Most women maintain their ability to breastfeed since only a few incisions are made in the glandular substance of the breast.* This bit of information seemed promising.

There is no guarantee—always the disclaimer—*but breastfeeding shouldn't be a problem.* And I believed. Or had I listened selectively? Did I think I heard a yes because they didn't tell me no?

After my trouble breastfeeding Zoey, I would return to my research and learn that the breast lift may have damaged my milk ducts, and as a result my milk supply suffered. But, sitting on the plastic surgeon's examination table, with a before-and-after-surgery photo album sitting on my knees, I didn't know about that. After assessing headless Polaroids featuring sad, tubular "before" breasts and the pert and springy orbs as pictured in the "after" shots, I was sold. I had my breast-lift surgery six weeks later and the operation was a success. My new breasts were proud specimens, high and tight and spherically sound. They may not have been perfect, but they looked perfect to me.

*   *

After Brenda places her on the scale, Zoey's peachy body curls into the fetal position, and she blinks warily against the brightness of morning. Watching Zoey lie there, totally vulnerable in her nakedness, stirs within me a consuming sadness. The guilt and self-doubt creep in. Somehow I've managed to screw this thing up. She is helpless without me, and yet I'm ill equipped to take care of her basic needs.

Brenda and I watch as the dial bounces around on the scale, begins to hover, then finally settles on a number. The baby has lost more weight. She hasn't regained her initial post-birth weight loss, and she's lost a few additional ounces. The scale appears to confirm my fear that my baby isn't getting enough to eat.

Zoey's tight fists go herky-jerky and she begins to make the fussing, wind-up noises that sound like a sneezing cat. Before she starts crying, I rescue her from the cool metal of the scale and place her to my breast, comforting her, for this moment. Zoey's weight loss prompts me to make another visit to the pediatrician. At the office we will discuss the baby's weight and consider our options. We will talk about supplementing.

What I don't know but will learn very quickly is that my breasts will soon become irrelevant to Zoey. Soon she won't want to work so hard at my breast for the little bit she can get, when the bottle feeds her so readily. She will try to nurse, then arch her back and refuse to latch on. Too quickly she will reject my breast altogether, my milk having failed her. Soon I will be the mother at the play date guiltily ladling scoopfuls of formula into a bottle.

Brian, Zoey, and I return from the pediatrician's office with a plan to begin supplementing. My worst fears are confirmed: I've been starving Zoey. Brian counters my statement with an eye roll—I'm hormonal and hyperbolic—but my anxiety persists. I can't help but categorize myself as the worst type of mother there is, the ignorant kind. How could I have not known? How could I have forced my pathetically meager supply of breast milk on her? No wonder she screamed all hours of the day. She was hungry. "Don't blame yourself," Brian tells me. "You didn't know."

But I should have known, or figured it out sooner. "That's all behind us now," Brian answers. "Let's move on."

And so we do. As I handle the weighty metal containers of premixed Enfamil in the baby aisle at Target, I recognize my karmic moment of reckoning. Here I am, the haughty breast-feeding advocate, gone over to the dark side of canned formulas. I will have to reevaluate my position on the breast-versus-formula debate and will learn to redefine what it means to successfully nourish my child.

At home I prepare the formula and feed Zoey her first bottle. She drains it, stopping only when I interrupt the feeding to burp her. Brian changes her diaper, swaddles her, and positions her in the bassinet. Zoey blinks and stares, and then fades easily into what will be her longest nap yet. We are stunned. She's not crying.

After an hour of silence, Brian and I go into the bedroom to check on the baby, sure that something is wrong. We approach Zoey's bassinet with anticipatory fear—the quiet is so profound that it seems to be ringing in my ears—and find our daughter sleeping soundly, her chest rising and falling evenly. Brian puts his arm around my shoulder and squeezes me. "I'm sure if she could talk to us right now she'd say thank you," he whispers.

I nod. And if Zoey could hear me right now, I would tell her that I'm sorry.

✳

Stephanie Kilroy graduated from the University of California, Los Angeles, with a degree in history. She also studied creative writing, and one of her plays, *Junk Hungry*, was produced in Los Angeles. She writes in Reno, Nevada, where she lives with her husband, Brian, and her four children, Leilani, Zoey-Cate, Leo, and Dominic.

WE'RE ALL IN THIS TOGETHER

Dana Sullivan

I'm a fairly competitive person. I'll admit it. Throw down a challenge, and chances are I'm in. There's one exception: parenting. Being a mother has been an extraordinarily humbling experience for me. And judging my fellow mothers isn't a sport I care to engage in. There are exceptions, of course. Leave a gun in your nightstand drawer—yes, I have a friend who did that—and you'll get an earful. Hold your baby on your lap while you're a passenger in a car—yep, I have a friend who did this, too—and your eyes will glaze over during my recitation of car crash statistics. But short of safety matters, I try to keep my mouth shut. I'm fumbling along just like everyone else; I'll admit that, too. Often I wonder: We're all in this together, so why are some women so bitchy?

The sniping starts before our babies are even born, sometimes from the most surprising sources. Take childbirth education classes, for instance. When my husband and I took ours, we "graduated" feeling like the biggest losers because we were having our baby in the hospital instead of at home or at a midwife-run birth center. This judgment was conferred upon us—albeit subtly—by the other parents-to-be in the group and also, not so subtly, by the registered nurse–midwife who taught our class. And yet this woman turned out to be one of the nurses caring for our son a month later while he was on life support, recovering from meconium aspiration syndrome following an emergency c-section. Surely she knew that sometimes things go wrong, even after a healthy pregnancy?

Then there was childbirth itself. I've had three cesareans. The first was a life-or-death situation; in fact, our son was several weeks old before we knew he'd live. My next two babies were delivered at thirty-six weeks because of various complications. And yet on more than one occasion I've had to defend the need for my babies' "medical" births. I've listened to at least a dozen women opine how their children's "natural" (that is, drug-free) births—either in a hospital or at home—somehow made their birth experiences more significant than mine. They have suggested that their experiences have actually made them better mothers, because they were able to bond with their babies right away. My blood pressure rises just thinking about those encounters.

Which brings me to breastfeeding. I am a huge advocate of breastfeeding. So far, I have spent a total of five years nursing three babies. I have written at least a dozen how-to articles for various parenting magazines that, I hope, have helped some women get past the early, difficult days. I will go on and *on* about how much I loved breastfeeding to anyone who wants to listen. And yet . . . and yet, I would no more express my opinion that "breast is best" to someone who has not asked for it than I would tell a friend that her expensive, trendy jeans really highlight her muffin top. I just don't see the point of reciting the list of breastfeeding's benefits—in this day and age, who doesn't know them?—to someone who has decided that breastfeeding isn't for her.

But some of us aren't so reticent. I remember when a friend of mine decided a few days after her daughter's birth that breastfeeding was too much. Too much pain. Too much work. Just too much. So she stopped, and started pumping instead. (Talk about too much—pumping ten times a day is *hard*!) That lasted for about three weeks. But when my friend started mixing formula, she was nearly drowned by a tsunami of unsolicited advice. "You have to stick it out for at least six weeks," one friend told her. "Just get the bottles out of the house so you're not tempted," said another. Some of it was well-meaning, of course, but a lot of it was counsel barely concealed as criticism. Since I was pregnant with my first child, and had neither given birth nor nursed a baby, I could only listen and tell her what I truly believed: that only she knew what was best for her and her baby. I also recall thinking—as I listened to my friend so obviously in distress, describing her scabby breasts and the bloody milk that her daughter was spitting up, all the while getting zero support from her husband—I'd reach for the bottle, too.

I know of one first-time mom who weaned her daughter at three months for a host of reasons, one of which was her baby's failure to thrive. She soon became reluctant to leave the house, because when she was out and about she was accosted one too many times by other mothers, complete strangers who would approach her when they saw her feeding her baby from a bottle. "Why are you using formula?" or "Don't you know that breastfeeding is the best thing you can do for your baby?" they would ask, with barely disguised disdain. When Rebecca had twins two years later, she decided to bottle-feed from day one.

"My daughter was healthy and happy, even though I had weaned her at three months, and I just couldn't go through the drama again," she said. (Interestingly, no one pestered her about her decision not to nurse the twins.)

How about the women who proudly proclaim that they *exclusively* breastfed for six months or twelve—"because, you know, it's what the American Academy of Pediatrics recommends." As if anyone who doesn't follow the AAP's recommendation is a fool. Or worse: negligent.

I even have a friend, I'll call her Mary, who came to pick me up for a movie one night and saw me preparing a bottle for my then six-month-old. She immediately shared this with me: "My babies have never had that *poison*." Now, without getting too defensive, let me say that I reserved formula for rare occasions—having spent several months pumping milk when my premature or otherwise ill babies couldn't suckle made me really loathe pumping once they finally latched on—but I was so shocked by her comment that I sputtered something defensive when I should have just told her to piss off. I'm still friends with Mary. But I haven't forgotten that incident. (Sometimes when I'm at her house and I see the smorgasbord of snacks laden with high-fructose corn syrup in the pantry, I really have to hold my tongue. I want to point out that while her kids may have been *exclusively* breastfed for *twelve months*, surely she negates all those benefits with the toxic junk she plies her kids with every day. . . . Oops. Now there *I* go.)

Why do we do this to each other? My theory is that we're so insecure we just can't help ourselves. Little more than a generation ago it was almost a given that a woman would stop working, at least for several years, to stay home and raise children. And since women in our mothers' generation followed their doctors' orders when it came to feeding with breast or bottle, it wasn't a matter that was up for discussion. Nor was it something that our mothers criticized one another about. Today some of us have the option to work or stay home—or to do some combination of both—and I think that having choices has made us defensive about all of them. We haven't figured out how to live and let live.

From what I can tell, men aren't as critical. Sure, they might harass one another about a lame jump shot, or bad taste in music. But I can no sooner imagine my husband inquiring about whether a friend's baby gets breast milk or formula—and then offering his opinion about whether the friend is making a good or bad choice—than I can imagine him making the case for homemade baby food versus jarred. These scenarios are as far-fetched as his asking me if his jeans make his butt look big.

I'm tired of it. Whether a woman has an epidural or delivers her babies without medication, whether she works or stays home, has babysitting help or does it all herself, feeds her babies from the breast or bottle or both, it's *all* challenging. I truly believe that we are all doing our best to love our children the best way we know how. What if we made a collective vow to cut each other some slack? Since we're all in this together, let's all just lighten up.

✳

Dana Sullivan has written for *The New York Times*, *O: The Oprah Magazine*, *Real Simple*, *More*, *Outside*, *Self*, *Health*, *Parenting*, and *Parents*, among other publications.

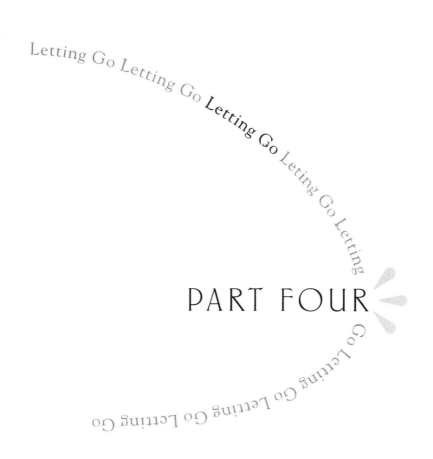

Letting Go Letting Go Letting Go Letting Go Letting Go Letting Go Letting Go Letting Go Letting Go

PART FOUR

THE BOYS WHO NURSED FOREVER

Fernanda Moore

Nothing I've ever held in my arms is more lovely than a contentedly nursing baby—that exquisite rosebud mouth, those drowsy eyes, those delicious flushed cheeks, chubby fingers clutching my hand, the slow rhythm of the baby sucking. Life is often hectic and noisy; nursing never is. Still, it's disconcerting when the baby, without warning, suddenly unlatches and sits up.

"Mom," he says.

"Yeah?" I answer.

"You know when things fall down to the ground?"

"Yeah," I say.

"That's called gravity."

My mother, who unfortunately happens to be both in town and in the room, snorts loudly. The little nursling snuggles down and turns with a sigh back to my breast. And I find myself wondering for the umpteenth time: How did those other mothers, the ones whose kids now have for their nocturnal joneses sippy cups, thumb-sucking habits, or complicated, fraught relationships with their pacifiers, manage? How, exactly, does one kick the nursing habit?

I have two sons: Zander, who turns ten this year, and Thad, who is three and a half. The former nursed until he was four, and the latter, not to be oedipally outdone, is still at it. (Ask him, sometime when the nipple is in his mouth, when he plans to quit, and he'll casually hold up four fingers.) This has caused tremendous consternation among my friends and family, all of whom think any child capable of walking over and unbuttoning your shirt (not to mention discussing Newtonian physics while *in flagrante*) is much too old to be nursing. In short, they think I'm crazy. And, in a way—in several ways, actually—I see their point.

All narratives of tragic debauchery begin the same way—but listen. I truly never thought it would happen to me.

When I was pregnant, I figured I'd give breastfeeding the old college try. Everyone said it was best for the baby, and besides, my own mother (who'd fed me formula—"You refused my breast! I worried you'd starve!"—but happily nursed my younger sister and brother) had only good things to say about the experience. "There's nothing like it," she told me over and over again. "When the baby suddenly looks up at you, and then unlatches to give you a big, milky grin? Well, it's just the most amazing thing." Bottle feeding, on the other hand, was a different matter. "What a nightmare." She shuddered. Feeding me, apparently, wasn't milky grins and the blissful union of mother and child, but endless sterilization of rubber nipples, boiling of bottles, measuring and mixing and pouring, getting up in the middle of the night and going down to the freezing kitchen (I was born in February). All that—coupled with a vaguely alarming story about how my father forgot to feed me, or dropped me, or dropped the bottle, or something (the conversation always devolved into politics at that point, so I never got the full story) the night Bobby Kennedy was shot—and I was completely sold. Give me a milky, loving grin over the horror of rubber nipples. Plus, the idea of actually sterilizing anything in my kitchen was improbable, to say the least.

The day Zander was born he nursed for five straight hours while I, blissed out on oxytocin, watched the Oscars on the hospital television. Every so often a nurse stuck her head in the door, ordered me to desist ("Ten minutes per side, or your nipples will get fatigued!"), and departed, shaking her head. I ignored her. My nipples, I felt, were not a topic for polite conversation, and besides, the baby was quiet—what was her problem? Eventually we snuggled down, eschewing the handy bassinet next to the bed, and dozed and nursed until the sun rose. The nurses weren't speaking to us the next morning, though they did slam a free Enfamil sample on top of my diaper bag as we left.

In the weeks that followed, the baby and I developed a perfect routine. He nursed. I read, stared out the window, chatted on the phone, gazed happily at his fuzzy little head. We slept, if you could call it sleeping, side by side. In the manner of hospital nurses, relatives came and went, offering advice, which I treated like a can of Enfamil. After several months, the advice gained focus and intent. Breastfeeding, the relatives chanted, ties you down. It alienates kind, eager-to-baby-sit relations, keeps you up at night, makes your kids too dependent, turns them gay, guarantees they'll . . . wait, I'm getting ahead of myself. Anyway, the relatives agreed, breastfeeding ties you down.

If, however, you have nothing in particular to be tied down *from*—if, say, you're an aimless fourth-year graduate student with a kid who's happiest when he's latched on, plus a chronic disinclination to fix supper, breastfeeding turns out to be the very thing. Oh, I was smug about it. Nursing, I told the relatives, dovetailed perfectly with Zander's and my temperaments—why, it was like falling off a log! "Right," my mother said, sometime after Zander turned two. "But you know, we all figured you'd climb back *on* the log at some point." On cue, Zander ambled over and tugged at my sweater. My mother rolled her eyes in disgust. "Charles Lindbergh's mother followed him to college. They were *roommates*," she said darkly.

Breastfeeding these days is hardly a radical act—for every old lady who gives you the fishy eyeball when you whip it out in public for your six-month-old, there are two million legal, moral, and scientific endorsements of your right—nay, duty!—to feed your baby wherever you please. I was always shameless about public nursing, but by the time Zander turned three, my sang-froid was diminishing. The playgrounds we frequented were lousy with ideology-addled parents, each more vocal than the last, but they'd shut right up about their hemp diaper covers when Zander sprinted over from the sandbox to request a few minutes under my shirt. As fun as it was to be subversive, even I felt a little squeamish when I realized I had, for two whole years, been nursing someone with *shoes*. And *teeth*.

What I needed was a like-minded, milky support group, and I found it in La Leche League. La Leche League's many detractors claim it's full of cultish nursing imperialists who run around ferreting out bottle-fed babies, the better to shame their mothers. This may be true, though I never saw any evidence of it. I showed up at my first meeting because I figured it was the only place on the planet I could confess I'd offered to let Zander nurse for five extra minutes if he properly used the big toilet, and I was right. "Wow, what a great idea," someone said. "Much healthier than M&Ms." I sighed happily. At La Leche League, I was mainstream again.

At every meeting we went around the room, sharing little anecdotes. It was a badge of honor to nurse one's older kids all through pregnancy till the new baby was born. There were, apparently, herbal remedies for sore nipples in the first trimester, plus heartwarming tales of sibling bonding as each child snuggled up to a breast of her own. Nursing twins was ho-hum; triplets were feasible, adopted babies were admirable, secondgraders were not unusual. Man, I thought, unhooking my bra. These people were *weird*.

Only problem was, you couldn't really get much solid advice on weaning. It wasn't a taboo subject, per se—as far as I could tell, it just wasn't *done*. There were a couple of books with *weaning* and *toddler* in their titles lying around La Library—I snatched them up—but even the books seemed baffled. You might try reading a story or offering a cup of juice when your child wants to nurse, they said weakly. If that doesn't work—well! Certainly he'll stop nursing by college! (And if not, he'll fly solo across the Atlantic, I thought. Take heart!)

When Zander was three and a half and still nursing morning and naptime and bedtime and in between if he stubbed his toe or got upset or overtired or something, my husband was invited to a conference in Italy. I was dying to go with him, and even though we could afford only one extra plane ticket, it never occurred to me not to take Zander along. If he scrunched up a little and breastfed conspicuously at the gate, I figured, he could easily pass for under two. And if I could somehow keep him from *talking* for the nine-hour flight, he'd make a swell stowaway.

But my mother-in-law craftily offered to baby-sit, and somehow I was swayed. Before I knew what was happening, we were blowing kisses at the airport and heading off for eight whole days. And then I was wandering around Lake Como, almost hallucinating with the forgotten joy of being alone—not to mention the forgotten joy of having handsome Italians drive their Vespas onto the sidewalk, the better to ogle my suddenly magnificent rack. After seventeen suckle-free hours, I had, as the French say, the whole world in my balcony. And my child—whom I missed in an absent-minded way, but who was, I realized, hardly the most erotic accessory—was, when we finally called to check, as happy as a clam.

In the week that followed, I spent the days checking out my cleavage in the windows of parked Fiats, and the nights gingerly massaging my dripping breasts over our hotel sink. The potentially tragic symbolism (all that lovely milk down the drain!) didn't bother me in the least. Zander who? Hey, nursing ties you down! My only regret was the time I'd wasted reading those stupid books on weaning, neither of which mentioned the fail-safe Italian holiday cure.

Alas, some bonds transcend time and distance. The minute we got back, though Zander hadn't clawed at my mother-in-law's bosom even once, the whole damned racket started up again. It didn't last forever, of course (the books were right about that). In the end, Zander took leave of breastfeeding so subtly and unremarkably that neither I nor any of my nosy relatives quite realized what had happened until it was over. I do know he persisted for at least another six months, since I distinctly remember feeling a bit of the old subversive frisson at the thought that I was nursing an actual four-year-old. Yet despite everyone's dire predictions, he seems to have come through the whole experience without any obvious psychological scars. (Okay, so he did go through a fairly vehement cross-dressing phase right around weaning, but I'm sure that was just a coincidence.)

With Thad, I'm either more laid-back or more beaten down. Without meaning to, I've been pegging his tenure at the breast to a friend's weaning trajectory; when her son, who's half a year older, a head taller, and about fifteen pounds heavier than Thad, finally hangs it up, I figure I've got a six-month grace period before my kid becomes the Oldest Nursing Boy in Town. We even invented a charming little poem, which our children obediently recite: "When you're four, there's no more." Whether it will work better than a story, a cup of juice, or a week in Italy *senza bambini* is anyone's guess.

In darker moments I've feared that my indolence and Thad's persistence might prolong our milky symbiosis until even La Leche League gives us the boot. Possibly I should get a job—if the enforced separation doesn't hasten things along, I can use my salary to endow a Charles Lindbergh Mother-Son Dormitory wherever Thad decides to attend college. Or maybe we should do something more vivid with our afternoons, instead of nursing, reading, and (inevitably) napping till Zander gets home from school. But then I remember that Zander simply quit one day, and his little brother seems determined to imitate him in everything. And while there are plenty of pangs every mother experiences as her babies grow up, I promise that if your kid nurses until he cuts off the circulation to your legs when he lies across your lap, weaning, when it occurs, comes as a happy relief.

✳

Fernanda Moore has written for numerous publications, including *New York Magazine*, *The New York Times Magazine*, and *Parenting*, and she is a regular book reviewer for the *Nashville Scene*. She lives with her family in Swarthmore, Pennsylvania.

MOM AND MACHINE

Maura Rhodes

Not long ago I took a big shopping bag full of outgrown clothing to a children's consignment store called Milk Money. In the bag were pint-sized sweaters and tiny dresses, a plush red snowsuit that all four of my children wore as infants, miniature slippers in the shape of cowboy boots that I could no longer squeeze over my toddler's toes. Because the store deals in baby gear, I also brought along a few bright-colored plastic toys that no one played with anymore, and a breast pump that I had recently retired, when said toddler turned one.

The clothing, the toys, all stayed at the store, awaiting a new life in someone else's closet or playroom. The breast pump, however, came back home with me. It wasn't that the owner of the store turned down the pump. In fact, she was eager to add it to the corner where she stocks maternity frocks and baby-name books. With her keen eye for all things resaleable, she saw that the pump was in excellent condition. Plus, it was something she could price at more than eight or ten bucks.

It wasn't that, even though the pump would be one of the higher-ticket items in the store, it would still go for a mere $75, when originally it cost over $300. I understood that this was a used-clothing shop, where people come to score bargains.

It wasn't that somewhere deep down I thought I might need the pump again. Despite my not-so-secret desire for "just one more baby" (this is the part where my friends will roll their eyes; my oldest, who's seventeen, is going off to college next year!), the odds are against that happening.

Now you may be wondering why in the name of Hera, the Greek goddess of motherhood, I'd cling to a contraption that's in some ways a torture device for the mammaries. After all, pumping is nothing like nursing an infant. No rosebud lips latched on to your nipple. No starfish hands kneading your breast. No seven pounds of warm, delicious heft burrito-ed in a soft blanket to cradle. No satisfied, satisfying gulping to tell you that what you're doing, right at this minute, is one of the most important things you'll ever do in your life. If you've ever used a pump yourself, or seen one in use (which in some ways is worse, I suspect), you know what I'm talking about. Pumping is to breastfeeding as a vibrator is to making love: a mechanical substitute that gets the job done all right, but without the love part.

And yet, I seem to be attached to my breast pump in a weirdly emotional way. In the weeks since my visit to the ironically named Milk Money, the pump has sat in a corner of my bedroom, prompting me on occasion to contemplate its strange hold on me. And somehow, between reading board books, checking homework, signing field trip slips, wiping noses, wiping bottoms, and wiping tears (not to mention juggling my own work deadlines), I think I've figured it out. My breast pump is a symbol that even as a working mom, I'm a good mom.

It's like this: I worked throughout all of my pregnancies and went back full time at the end of each maternity leave. When my first baby (Will, the seventeen-year-old) was born, I had every intention of breastfeeding when I was home—mornings, nights, and weekends—and keeping up a supply of pumped milk for when I was at the office. Here's how my first day back on the job after having Will turned out:

At around three in the afternoon, the phone rings. It's Will's nanny, Thelma. "You need to come home right away. Your baby's very hungry."

"Oh, no, there's plenty of milk in the freezer," I say. Had I actually forgotten to show her my stash?

"He drank it all."

He drank it all. It's just four words, but they're packed with meaning. What Thelma's telling me is that every pearly drop of milk coaxed from my breasts over the past few weeks, decanted carefully into tiny plastic bags and festooned with red twist ties, is gone.

"I'll take the next train," I say, glancing at the schedule and trying to calculate how long it'll actually take me to get home, tear open my shirt, and relieve my starving baby.

"He can't wait," says Thelma. "I'll have to buy formula."

I wince. Will's screaming right into the phone. I guess Thelma's holding him near the receiver now (to comfort him? to make a point?). "There's cash in my top dresser drawer," I tell her. I hang up and burst into tears.

So much for the best-laid plans of mice and moms. That fateful phone call was the beginning of the end of nursing my son. Even though I was producing plenty of milk to sustain him when I was with him, and was able, with my dinky little battery-powered pump, to set aside a few bottles when I wasn't, the wholesale disappearance of my initial cache of milk set me back enough that I was never able to catch up completely (or didn't have the energy to try), and so Thelma was supplementing with formula daily. Feeling defeated, kind of like when you get that first ding in a new car and say to yourself, "What the hell, why bother?" and start letting your coffee slosh on the upholstery and the kids eat whatever crumbly crap they want to in the back seat, I weaned Will from my still highly productive breasts when he was six months old.

Seven years later, I got pregnant with my second child. A lot had changed by that time: Will's dad and I had split up, I'd remarried, and I'd started working as an editor at a parenting magazine. I share that detail in particular because at my new job I received firsthand, from those eager PR folks at the many research labs doing breastfeeding studies, a steady stream of press releases heralding each new finding and urging me, as a journalist, to get the word out: Nursing staves off ear infections. It prevents obesity. It promotes bonding. It makes babies smarter. It lowers the risk of sudden infant death syndrome. It's a matter of life and death.

The effect that the brouhaha over breastfeeding had on me was twofold. First, there was panic: The American Academy of Pediatrics was now recommending that, if at all possible, infants be nursed for at least a year. What had I done to my son by cutting off his milk supply when we were only halfway there? Was I to blame for Will's chronic ear infections? As a first-grader he was still sporting ear tubes—his second set! And recently he'd become so fearful of letting me out of his sight that he would follow me five steps to answer the door. Was his anxious attachment some manifestation of my having put a bottle between his flesh and mine when he was still an infant?

Second, there was determination. I vowed that the baby I

was now carrying would never so much as taste a drop of formula. I would do as the AAP said and nurse my baby for a year, and after that for as long as she wanted, whenever she wanted, between her meals of toddler mush and cow's milk. (Or until she got old enough to talk; I wasn't interested in breastfeeding a preschooler who might pipe up in public and ask for some "booby.") And as my daughter swam blithely in her own private ocean, my resolve to be the sole provider of her nutrition was growing apace with her sprouting fingers and toes and eyelashes, hurtling towards something bordering on fanaticism.

To cut to the chase: Eliza was born, and yes, I managed to avoid giving her formula for her first year, despite going back to work when she was three months old. The same was true of Lucas and Wyatt, babies number three and four. And this collective accomplishment, I understand, was at the root of my love affair with my breast pump.

The pump entered my life when Eliza was just days old and my milk came in with a vengeance, leaving me so engorged that she couldn't latch on, much less empty my rock-hard breasts. I sent my husband out to buy the most powerful pump he could find, and my new, souped-up machine had me on the first *th-rump th-rump*: It could suck circles around the wimpy pump I'd had when Will was a baby. I was de-engorged in no time and had my first batch of milk for the freezer. For the rest of my maternity leave, even after Eliza nursed to bursting, the pump could still extract a few ounces to be set aside. And when I went back to work, my thrice-daily pumping sessions were efficient and productive. Because the pump was not only powerful but designed to empty two breasts at once, I quickly figured out how to hold both funnels in place with one hand and answer emails or edit manuscripts with the other. I could feed my baby and earn my paycheck all at the same time—the modern, maternal equivalent of bringing home the bacon and frying it up in the pan!

The pump's portability and discreet design (when not in use, it looks like a chic black backpack, not a lactation aid) also served me well. I was never shy about breastfeeding my babies whenever and wherever they demanded a snack: restaurants, parties, nail salons mid-pedicure. With my pump I could, and did, empty my breasts in unlikely places as well: in a public restroom in Philadelphia while on a field trip with Will's sixth-grade social studies class; during an overnight business trip to Washington, DC, when I stored the pumped milk in the ice bucket in my hotel room, getting up to replenish the ice during the night.

Was I a little nuts? Maybe. Was my obsession driven purely by the resounding reports that breast is best? Absolutely not. Sure, the research findings nagged at me. (Although I got over my initial worries that I had set Will up for a lifetime of illness and insecurity by weaning him: He got ear infections because he was prone to them; his sudden-onset separation anxiety coincided with my remarriage and the impending birth of his baby sister.) But the roots of my obsession went deeper, to the very core of what being a good mom, in spite of being a working mom, means, at least for me.

Most any woman who chooses, or has, to work after having kids will tell you that no matter how much she likes her job (and I truly loved mine), the motherhood-career combo can be fraught with guilt. It necessitates leaving your children to be cared for by someone who isn't you. Each day that you put on grownup clothes and walk out the door you feel as if you're abandoning your child anew. That, at least, was my experience.

By not being with my babies 24/7, I felt guilty, and sad, and even to some degree like a lousy mom. Every time I shut the door to my office and hooked up my pump, though, a little bit of the guilt and sorrow drained away. With every yellow-capped bottle of milk that I tucked into a corner of the office fridge, the longing that I felt for the infant at home was assuaged. With the help of my breast pump, what I couldn't give my babies in minutes and hours of time, I could make up for in ounces and ounces of milk.

So now that I've teased out the complexities of my relationship with my breast pump, what will become of it? The next time I have a bag full of too-small clothing to take to Milk Money, I'll bring the pump along and leave it. I don't need it around anymore. I have my beautiful children—Will, my college-bound almost-man; Eliza, my eight-year-old writer and fashion-model-to-be; Lucas, my five-year-old musician and gourmand; and Wyatt, my all-boy toddler who needs a new pair of slippers—to remind me that I have been, and am, a good mom.

❊

Maura Rhodes is a contributing editor for *Parenting* magazine and the author of several books, including *Radu's Simply Fit*, with Radu Teodorescu, and *Baby Must-Haves: The Essential Guide to Everything from Cribs to Bibs*. Rhodes lives in Montclair, New Jersey, with her husband and four children.

MOTHER'S LITTLE HELPERS

Melisssa Balmain

Not long ago I had an ominous chat with my friend Mel, who was in the midst of weaning her third kid.

"My hormones are changing," she groaned. "My real personality is coming back!"

Even as I assured her that I love her real personality, which I do, I could feel my shoulders knotting up. Soon I'd have to wean a kid, too—my second-born, Lily, then fourteen months old. And I looked forward to the experience about as much as a junkie looks forward to rehab.

My favorite thing about breastfeeding, after all, is that it gives you free, safe, and legal access to mood-altering drugs. So what if you haven't slept in twenty-four hours? Who cares if your hair hasn't been washed in seventy-two? What's the big deal if your house looks like the sale aisle at Kmart and your office looks even worse and you and your spouse just had a fight over how to clean the baby's neck folds? Just latch the kid on and in minutes you're floating on a mellow high, courtesy of mother's little helpers—prolactin, which makes milk, and oxytocin, which delivers it.

I also had un-favorite things about breastfeeding: plugged ducts, mastitis, babies chomping on me like lion cubs chomping on a wildebeest. But none of those made me want to actually quit.

Swacked on nursing hormones, I was more patient, more fun. I'd go from Joan Crawford to Donna Reed—game for hearing my then six-year-old, Davey, play the same note four hundred times on his accordion, then letting him "experiment" in the bathroom sink with my toothpaste. If the baby and I were alone in the house, I might drift into Cheech-like reverie, staring with happy stupidity at the whorls of her ear (was that the shape of a mermaid's tail? King Tut's head?). If I'd had a rough day, I might even become both pacifier and pacified by letting her nap while she nursed.

And there had been plenty of rough days during Lily's first fourteen months. First, I discovered that our house was swimming with radon gas. (On a whim I had gotten the levels rechecked, never imagining they had soared to Chernobyl heights since a test we'd done six years before.) Then fat black spiders with red hourglasses on their bellies began turning up in my living room. ("Yep," a cheery entomologist told me when I brought him one in a baby-food jar. "That's a black widow, all right.") Then, most alarming of all, Lily started gaining less and less weight and dropped lower and lower on the pediatric weight chart until she fell right off the bottom.

Normally, any one of these crises would have turned me into a complete wreck. Under the influence of breastfeeding, though, I was only a semi-wreck. While I did worry that my family would get lung cancer from the radon, I also managed to convince myself—based on research—that this was unlikely, given our length and degree of exposure. I vetted radon-mitigation companies, chose one, and had a man dig under our basement and install the world's priciest fan.

I shuddered when the entomologist suggested I roam our house with a flashlight to hunt for more black widows. But then I took a breath and roamed. Luckily, the first spiders I had found seemed to be all there were—unless you count the untold millions that, according to the radon guy, had colonized the crawlspace below our living room.

As for the Incredible Shrinking Baby, I admit I went ever so slightly off the deep end. Still, even as I obsessed over calories and doctor's scales and the chances that Lily might have cystic fibrosis (genes for it run in our family), I managed to stay more or less functional. I confirmed, with help from a lactation consultant, that Lily was getting enough to eat. I told myself over and over that our pediatrician was right: My daughter—bright, active, clear-lunged—was probably just small, not sick. And I didn't cry until the last in a long string of tests came back negative and I could collapse with relief.

Thank you, mother's little helpers.

"I think I'm addicted to oxytocin," I confessed to my husband, Bill, soon after Mel and I had our weaning talk.

"Well," he said, "that's better than being hooked on OxyContin."

But how much longer could I keep getting my fix? Week by week, Lily was losing interest in my boobs. Gone were the days when I could nurse her while yakking on the phone or reading Harry Potter books to Davey. Now we practically needed to be in a soundproof booth or she'd unlatch and sit up in a flash, eager for the real fun to begin.

For a couple of months more, I persevered. "Still going?" Mel asked in Lily's sixteenth month, sounding a tad wistful.

"Still going—sort of."

Lily had been letting me know, none too subtly, that she was ready to move on. While nursing, she dug her fingernails into the back of my hand. After draining breast A, her way of declining breast B was to smack me in the face. We began dropping feedings. Goodbye, tipsy evenings. So long, stoned afternoons. One day in her seventeenth month, it was finally time to go cold turkey.

Lily didn't seem to mind when, instead of breastfeeding her that morning, I simply scooped her up and trotted into the kitchen to pack Davey's lunch. I felt a bit insulted. (*I've made five hundred quarts of milk for you, and this is the thanks I get?*) But the truth is, for a short while afterwards, I didn't mind much either. I even celebrated the fact that, once again, I could eat garlic with impunity.

Then, just like Mel, I noticed my real personality returning. First came my Chicken Little, blow-things-out-of-proportion side—the side that turned the firing of a new babysitter into a guilt-ridden weep fest.

"The woman's probably forgotten all about it by now," Bill consoled me, as I broke down yet again, a week after canning her.

"I know!" I wailed. "But you should have seen her face when I told her. She's such a sweet person. If only she weren't so *incompetent*."

And I sobbed some more.

Nighttime brought slim relief. Lily's disdain for breast milk notwithstanding, she refused to quit her old nursing schedule and continued to wake—and wake her parents—in the wee hours. A hug or two sent her right back to Dreamland. I, meanwhile, was left banging on its gates until dawn; how had I not realized, during all those months, that nursing was my key to unconsciousness? Fifteen minutes or so after I finally conked out, Bill and I would be awakened by Lily *and* her brother, who climbed into our bed and bounced around while we tried to shield our kidneys from their kid knees. My eyes burned. My head throbbed. My short-term memory vanished faster than you can say, "Where the #@%# did I put my shoes?" God, how I longed for just one tiny hormonal hit.

Rocking with Lily in the chair where we used to nurse, reading or playing peekaboo instead, was great, but it wasn't enough. I began eating more chocolate (or, as I came to think of it, methadone for recovering breastfeeders). A few months before Lily turned two, I tried to boost my endorphins—and shrink my choco-padded gut—by walking more and taking up Pilates. I started to feel better.

Then Joan Crawford came roaring back, worse than she'd ever been—even counting the time in Lily's third month when I'd caught Davey teaching her, not gently, how to do karate.

Now I found myself snapping at my son every day. Forget accordion music and Crest experiments. His mere voice had become more than I could take. "Stop talking!" I was horrified to hear myself say, when he had been monologuing about Lord Voldemort, or Jacob Two-Two, or his undying quest for a Toy That Can Do Everything. "Just be quiet for five minutes, okay? Mommy needs a rest."

I was sure I hadn't been half as rotten after weaning Davey. I had felt withdrawal pangs, yes, but not this prickliness, this intolerance, which boiled over no matter how hard I tried to recapture my inner 1950s-sitcom mom. When I confessed my hideous behavior to friends, most just smiled knowingly. "Welcome to life with two kids," they said. "Don't worry—it gets easier." But *when*?

After Lily turned two, Joan showed up even more often—an equal-opportunity shrew now that my daughter had hit the age of tantrums and tyranny. "Stop throwing Mr. Potato Head in the dishwasher!" I barked at Lily, forgetting all about the art of sly distraction. "No, I cannot read you *Arthur's Underwear* while I'm driving!"

How was it, I wondered, that the pharmaceutical giants had yet to market nursing hormones to post-weaning moms? I bet they'd sell at least as well as Viagra. And how come—here was an idea—dairies didn't slip a few cc's of them into specially marked cartons of skim? Surely they had plenty on hand, given all the hormones they were pumping into their cows. I did eventually find something online called OxyCalm, a vanilla-scented, non-FDA-approved nasal spray containing "a very dilute solution of Oxytocin." "Helps promote relaxation, improve mood, and enhance inner peace and tranquility," the website declared. "Try it as a safe alternative to smoking." I imagined trying it myself, every three minutes or so, as an alternative to Chicken Little and Ms. Crawford. Still, I didn't dare buy any. Who knew what side effects this stuff had, or if it even worked? Despite my oxy-jonesing, I was terrified of actual drug abuse—and had been ever since reading a scared-straight-type book in seventh grade.

For now, I told Mel on the phone, the only remedy I could think of was to breastfeed a third child. "But we both know that's not happening," I added. I was old and fibroid-prone and besides, my tubes were tied.

Mel, whose own mood seemed to be on an upswing, suggested deep breathing. Also massage, meditation, and taking more time for myself. "I'm much nicer when I slow down," she said. "But there's no one solution."

A day or two after that, I woke with a start at 7:00 A.M. to realize that Lily, for maybe the first time all year, had slept straight through the night. Then both kids got in bed with Bill and me and began their usual routine of bouncing, poking, pinching, singing, shrieking, and kidney ramming.

"Good morning, good morning, good morning!" I said, hugging everybody.

Bill raised an eyebrow as if to ask, What's gotten into you?

"Sleep," I sighed. "Best damn drug of all."

᳂

Melissa Balmain's writing has appeared in *The New Yorker, The New York Times, Details,* and other magazines, newspapers, and anthologies. A contributing editor and humorist for *Parenting* and *Babytalk,* she's at work on several books.

WEAN

Catherine Newman

Day 1. After only a few tears and the brief pressing of her damp face to the damp front of my T-shirt, the baby is asleep. I run a bath, massage my lumpy, aching breasts under the hot water, and milk billows out like smoke, clouding the water before it disappears. By the time I wrap myself in a towel, my bosom is hanging down to my waist like a pair of empty feed sacks. I'm reminded suddenly of those statues of Romulus and Remus squatting under the wolf who nursed them, her long teats dangling down into their faces like banana peels.

Oh, this aching! Part body, part soul—like that feeling when a lover is on you, on you, on you, and then suddenly *gone*, and you're left holding a fragrant T-shirt to your nose, your body clenching around its own aloneness.

This poor baby: yoinked abruptly from the boob right before her second birthday, since I'm needing to take a strong antibiotic for a systemic infection. Weaning her older brother was easier. I got pregnant, and my milk turned thin and blue, like what my mother grew up drinking in a wartime convent boarding school in England: nothing fit for nourishing children.

With him, six long suckles a day dwindled first to four quick-
ies, and then to a bedtime and waking two, like a pair of milky
parentheses around the night. In the end there was just a single early-morning grazing of his mouth over my chest, like a
habit—the way a person might stroke his upper lip where a
mustache had once been. And then it was over and, save a discreet little hand up my shirt every now and then, there was
nothing left of our passionate and milky romance. Which was
just fine, what with the new baby and all. The boob-baton had
been perfectly handed off from one nursling to another.

But this, for me, is the last leg of this particular journey. I
don't plan to have any more children. My nursing days are of-
ficially over.

* * *

Day 2. I eat a can of tuna fish to celebrate—*Bring on the tox-
ins!*—and although I thought this would feel liberating, like a
silver (or mercury) lining, it doesn't. Instead I feel lonely, rat-
tling around in the empty apartment of my body, all by myself,
for the first time in six years. A friend once told us a story about
her toddler, shaking her head pityingly after she was weaned,
gesturing to her mother's body: "Now all you make in there is
pee and poop."

* * *

Day 10. I thought she was handling it so well, this baby—for
a week she patted my chest during the day, teasing, "What's
unda daya, Mama?" and cracking up into thick giggles. At bedtime she'd reach under my shirt with a doleful question—

"Messies?"—then she'd put her head on the mattress and go to sleep. But now it's taken a turn for the sad. She's two, but she's still such a baby, really, and discussions of nursing have been replaced by a nightly tantrum. One night it's because she wants to bounce on her brother's tummy during story time; another, it's because a string of malachite beads is just barely too short to fit over her head without being unclasped. She screams a terrible, high scream. She screams a wet, keening scream and sobs. She bites the sheet and then the mattress. She pulls Kleenex from the box and blots tragically at her own face. I sing her a favorite lullaby—"Shine shi-ine, shine shi-i-ine, moooooooon . . ."—and she snuffles, clambers into my arms finally, this giant baby. She says, "Can you wock me, Mama?" And I can. I do.

* *

Day 14. The two of us are in tears again. The baby's mouth is pulled into a sad shape, the corners pointed straight down like a miserable crescent moon, and she's hanging on to my front, pleading with me: "Just a *yitto*, Mama? A tiny sip?" By day she slurps water from a sippy cup, water from a melting ice cube, water from a revolting washcloth in her bath. But at night? At night she's like an addict, an addict who's losing it at a meeting, and she's had it with the grape juice, she's had it with the coffee. She just wants a real drink.

* *

Day 15. A confession: Now that she's not nursing at all, the baby is sleeping soundly through the night. I am better rested than I've been since the nineties. Who even knew I'd been so freaking tired?

∗   ∗

3 weeks. "Do you yike my messies?" We're naked, after a bath, and the baby is naming the parts of our bodies. She thrusts out her chest, points to the pale, pearly dots of her own nipples. She's not sad; she's chubby and damp and stopping to hammer out a happy tune on a rainbow-colored xylophone. But later the same afternoon she puts her head in my lap, sighs, and reaches up a melancholy hand to grope my boobs.

∗   ∗

4 weeks. It's Sunday morning: the post-bath naked-family rolling-around time. I've got a cup of tea that I'm trying to keep from spilling onto the bed. Over the course of an hour, the baby evolves towards being dressed: She's nude; she's got a robe; she's got a robe and a diaper. She pulls the comforter off my own naked chest, pokes each nipple in turn, announces a vague "Uh-oh!" Then she holds my jaw tenderly in her two hands, looks into my eyes like a teenaged boyfriend. "Can I do nurse?" she asks, and I say, "Okay." She puts her lips to my nipple and kisses it. Then she laughs and blows a raspberry. "Can I switch sides?" she asks, and I say, "Okay." Instead she pulls the comforter back up over my chest. Then she says fiercely, "No!" and yanks the covers back off. I think the technical name for this is *ambivalence*. Her face is strained wide with an unfamiliar, cocktail-party kind of smile that doesn't stretch all the way up to her sad eyes, and I feel heartbroken.

*   *

5 weeks. At a friend's house, where the baby is exhausted and miserable through dinner, I nurse her by accident. I'm talking to my friend, holding the baby while she cries, and then I'm hiking up my shirt. As soon as she latches on, I realize what I'm doing: her body goes heavy in my arms, and my eyes fill with tears. The only thing it's like is being reunited with a lover one last time. I stroke her hair; I try to memorize the gentleness of her face; I try to memorize the relaxed weight of her. Why is it like this? Why can't you spread out life's pleasures, not be so gluttonous? I have loved nursing, but I have not cherished it every single moment because, frankly, there's just been too much of it. I savor these last minutes with the baby, the baby who is disappearing even as I hold her.

*   *

2 months. The kids have the stomach flu. Every crack between every floorboard in the house has been barfed into. Every towel is soaking in the washing machine. Our comforter spins in the dryer and will never again be the same. And the worst of it? Her older brother at least sips wanly at his diluted juice, but the baby is sick and miserable, and, for the first time in her life, I have nothing to offer her. She pushes away the cup. I hold her in my arms, pressed against my dried-up chest, and I am sorry.

*   *

7 months. Pretend nursing has become our household's best joke. "Can I do nurse?" the baby asks now, and I say, "Sure!"

She raises her eyebrows comically, repeats, "*Sher?*" and I laugh. She pulls up my shirt, yanks down my bra, touches the tip of her tongue to each nipple, then skips away to her brother, screaming with laughter: "I did nurse!" I miss my old curvy self, my breasts that could have inspired the slogan Think Globally. But my libido—the one that's been cozily napping beneath bellies and boobs and hormones and babies—is waking up again. It's stretching, rubbing its eyes, and winking at my husband when he stands at the mirror to shave. When he looks at my breasts I do not even roll my eyes or say, "You have *got* to be kidding me." Still, I can't help feeling that you should be issued a new pair for the occasion: The segue from maternal lactating to manly fondling is just so awkward.

*   *

9 months. You know those men who loiter around while you're nursing at Barnes & Noble, hoping the baby might pull away so they can better leer at your milky gazongas? I'm like that. When friends nurse, I find myself staring from behind, all perverted-like. But I just want to see that doting little face looking up, the happy-fat cheeks, the roaming hand. Breastfeeding was such a lovely excuse for trading a fond gaze back and forth. Also for saying, "No biting!" or "All done!" or "Kill me—not again!" But for some reason that part seems to be evaporating, like mist, from the dreamy landscape of my nostalgia.

*   *

1 year. After the shower, one clear yellow drop beads up at the tip of each nipple. My poor body! Making milk on and on in this slight but adamant way. I feel sorry for it—the same way I feel about the insistent pangs of ovulation that nearly knock me over every month: Nobody thought to tell my ovaries that we're done having babies.

We're done having babies. Will I never again watch the pink moon of a nursing cheek, the eyelids sagging under the dead weight of lashes, the dopey, drooling grin of a milk-drunk baby? Will I never again reach across the night like a sleepy, gentle cow searching out her bleating calf? Will I never again rock a nursing baby into the sunrise, both of us brushed in Mary Cassatt peaches and pinks, like a timeless painting?

Life buzzes around me, and nostalgia must give way to the throb of the here and now. The baby stretches out on the bed, the brown of her curls reaching past her shoulders, the brown of her big eyes almost black. "Mom?" she says—she's experimenting, today, with calling me *Mom* instead of *Mama*— "Mom? Look at me." She pushes her fingers high over her head, points her toes as far down as they will go. "Mom, look. Look, Mom, I'm really growed up." And it's true. She is. And maybe I am, too.

※

Catherine Newman, author of the award-winning memoir *Waiting for Birdy*, is a contributing editor at *FamilyFun* and *Wondertime* magazines and a regular contributor to O: *The Oprah Magazine*. She lives in Massachusetts with her (entirely weaned) family.

WEANING ELLA

Jill Christman

My daughter, Ella, was just over two on the morning of her last breastfeeding. She'd stumbled in from her own room around 5:00 A.M., as usual, scrambled up into our bed, and latched on. Humming and suckling, she slipped into sweet sleep. Most mornings, this was the method by which my husband and I got to be those rare parents who sleep until eight.

This morning was different because I needed to catch a flight, without Ella, to interview job candidates for three days at the Modern Language Association conference in Washington, DC. I'd never been away from Ella for a night. Not ever. I lay awake and watched Ella nurse, feeling sick with love and the specter of our separation, touching the tiny droplets of sweat on her soft temple, watching her jaw pumping out the rhythm of our bodies together.

My husband, Mark, and I had decided that this forced separation would be the perfect weaning window, and I knew chances were good that this would be the last time she and I would lie together like this: cuddled, content, sleepy, and sleeping. I must have dozed off myself because the next thing I knew, the morning news was mumbling in my ear and the clock glowed 6:30. In that alarm-clock moment I did what I had always done when I needed to get up without Ella: I slipped my finger between her lips and my nipple to break the suction, then with gentle pressure held her under her chin until her sucking wound down and her mouth relaxed. And then I got out of the bed.

In the dark, on the way across the room to the shower, I realized what I had done. I had failed to mark the last time as the Last Time. Standing frozen in the warm stream of the shower, I felt as if that moment should have been something more. What should she and I have done? Lit a candle? Whispered a prayer? Shared a promise?

Think of all your last times in love. Did you know they were endings? The end? This time, so rare, I had known, and I had let it slip away.

On the plane to DC, my heart was breaking and my seat belt was broken. The buckle clicked, but when I leaned forward, the whole mechanism slid easily along the nylon strap. No resistance. No help at all in a crash, but then again, who survives an airplane crash? Nonetheless, I notified the flight attendant, who couldn't get the darn thing to clamp either, and then there we were, a whole planeful of people waiting on the tarmac because of my seat belt. I dismantled the thing and put it back together. It worked! The mechanics were canceled, we took off on schedule, and the flight attendant offered me a free drink for my heroism.

I didn't want to be on that plane. I wanted to see my baby. I ordered a Jack and Coke. Why the hell not? I wasn't nursing, after all. I wanted this high-noon cocktail to feel liberating. Instead, I deplaned with a big, fat headache.

We met with the job candidates in my gloomy hotel room. By day I dressed in a loose jacket to hide breasts that grew larger with every interview, and at night, when all of the candidates had gone, I peeled off my professor clothes and climbed naked, a mother again, into the shower. I needed to express milk—enough so I'd fit into my clothes, not enough to encourage production. *She's not here*, I told my body. *Give it up.*

Ba ba is our family word for breast milk. Months before I found myself in that dim hotel shower, wet and weeping, I read a sidebar in a parenting magazine that had made me smile. A recent study out of Australia reported that nursing toddlers say their mother's milk is "as good as chocolate" and "better than ice cream." No wonder Ella was crazy for *ba ba*. Sweet goodness and a cuddle with Mom. That's some soda fountain.

Standing under the warm stream, I lifted my hands up under my breasts, and they felt like full IV bags, liquid heft. What a waste to squeeze it all away, I thought, but I did. I did.

After three days in DC, I was afraid to go home. What would we be now?

On the plane I obsessed over our reunion, and all the possibilities scared me. Maybe she would run towards me, short arms flailing, demanding to be nursed. My husband and I had discussed this, of course, and he had been firm. He knows my weaknesses.

"You will say no," he told me on the phone. "You weren't here. It was hard. We're not going to do this to her again."

This made sense. But I wondered about the other end of the spectrum. *What if she's mad? What if she feels abandoned? What if she doesn't want to see me?*

When I pulled up in the car, Ella was waiting at the glass storm door, leaping intermittently. I watched her press her face and both palms against the glass and jump, a haze of breath and nose smear. From the driveway I could see she didn't plan to punish me for going away. Instead, she was all over me with hugs and stories. In those first happy hours, she said nothing of *ba ba*. I was enough.

But there was a bedtime ritual yet to be performed, and part of it was going to be missing.

After a bath with four rubber ducks, I dried her in the frog towel and got her into footie pajamas. My heart was in my throat. *Ba ba* time. "Hold me," Ella said. "Mommy, hold me."

"How about a *book?*" I said with forced cheer. "Do you want to read a book with Mommy on the couch? And then Daddy will read you some *more* books in the big-girl bed?" I heard the false notes ringing from my lips, and I knew she could, too. Ella's two, but she's no fool.

The book reading on the couch went fine: My *Opposites/Mis Opuestos*. "Ooh," I said. "Look! The green snake is lo-o-ong. *En español, largo*. Can you say *largo?*" Her pronunciation was surprisingly good. I sounded like a parody of a bedtime parent. When the book was finished, we headed back to the bedroom. I was as cheerful as Christmas morning, but Ella was on to me. She dug her heels into the area rug beneath the dining room table.

"I want some *ba ba*," she said. Mark and I made eye contact. This was what we'd been waiting for. "I want some *ba ba*."

I threw my head back and laughed (a friend of a friend had mentioned this technique and in this moment I had nothing better). "Oh no," I said, still laughing. "You don't want *ba ba*. You're a big girl!"

Mark repeated my message, smiling at Ella and then directing his expression to me and hissing, "Redirect! Redirect! Don't come in the bedroom. You'd better just stay out."

By now Ella was on the floor, sobbing. "But I *need ba ba*," she countered. "But I *need ba ba*." At this point nobody was saying anything just once.

I walked to a part of the house where I could not hear the screams. My breasts were aching. By the time I returned, maybe ten minutes later, the sounds were muffled. Reading sounds.

Mark appeared triumphant about an hour later, rubbing his eyes.

At seven the next morning, Ella scrambled up into our bed. She flopped on her belly and turned her face towards me, breathing softly. Her breath smelled like sweet corn. I fluffed a pillow to keep her head up with my head, not in the habitual place, breast side. I rubbed her back and hummed. This seemed to make her happy. But then she flopped around. "I need you to change my diaper," she said. "And then it will be seeping time."

I did. It was not sleeping time.

"I need Something," she said, capitalizing the *something* A. A. Milne–style.

Mark watched us through a cracked eye and chose this moment to intervene. "Do you want some water? In your sippy cup? Are you thirsty? Here you go." If he hadn't been supervising, would I have folded? Would it have been our little secret? I still wonder who was weaning whom.

Ella slapped the cup away. "No. I need *Something Else*." Amazing. She couldn't seem to remember what she wanted. She couldn't seem to remember what those dark, early-morning moments had been for throughout the first two years of her life. But we could see her mind working. Redirect. Redirect.

"I need *Something Else*."

Mark gave options. Juice, soymilk, Kix.

She rejected them all and turned to me, half remembering. "Roll over," she demanded. "Roll over."

Since I was facing her, I started to roll away, obediently, a woman without a plan. "Nooooooooooooooooooooo! Roll over! You need to open up the *ba bas*." She pulled on my heavy black shirt. "You need to open them up!"

And so it went—a cycle of remembering and forgetting until time did its work and made nursing a vestige of babyhood, an artifact, something that happened "last night" Ella's um brella term for all things gone by.

Later on the first full day of my return, Ella had seemingly forgotten about nursing again, and we made oatmeal cookies. After the margarine and the sugars, I reached up to turn on the KitchenAid, and, without being told, Ella put her hands flat on the countertop and said dutifully, "Only Mommy or Daddy can touch that machine." I wondered: If she can forget breastfeeding, the nearest and dearest thing she has known, after only five days, how can she remember anything at all? How can she hang on to something I've told her maybe twice about a mixer and not be cognizant of the soft keystone of her young life?

In the weeks after DC, even though I could reach out and touch her whenever I wanted, I missed Ella. I missed my baby. The relationship changed—it had to—once the nursing was over. I cuddled her, and she let me, but it wasn't the same. I had nothing to offer her that was mine and mine alone to give.

That can't be true, can it? It felt true.

We held back from each other, doing a kind of dance to avoid physical closeness that might remind us of what we once shared. I keep trying to figure out what this feeling was like—this stage on the letting-go continuum between giving birth and dropping her off for her first day of school—but since Ella is my first child,

I can compare this shift in intimacy only to the end of a romantic relationship. Not a messy, dirty breakup, but the kind born of time and change—the kind you both know has to come. Okay, so you talk and talk and talk. It's over. This is it. This is the best thing for everyone. But his stuff is still in your apartment, and he complains that the hide-a-bed couch is a back breaker. This is a time of transition. You agree he can stay for three more weeks until the lease starts on his new place. He can even sleep on his side of the bed, but he can't roll over onto your side.

But you know how many moles he has on his back. You know how he likes a swirl of honey in his coffee, but not the whole spoonful. You know he'll never replace the cap on the toothpaste, even if it's a flip-top designed for recalcitrants like him. You know everything. But you can't touch him when he's feeling sad about leaving. You can't, because if you do, well, there you go, you're back in it, and you'll both have to begin the separation all over again.

This is how Ella and I felt, and I know her well enough that I can speak for her, too. Here's the difference: She wasn't leaving. Not yet. For now, she wasn't going anywhere, and we needed to figure out what our new intimacy was going to look like. We needed to figure out what would replace what we'd lost, what we'd grown beyond. This was exhausting.

A week after my return, this involved a turkey and hummus sandwich, with the crusts cut off, at 3:30 A.M. A picnic. The next day I sighed and said to Ella's babysitter, "I don't want her to think that this is what we do—we wake up in the middle of the night and have picnics! But she was *hungry*. She ate the whole sandwich. I can't just let her be hungry."

The babysitter laughed. "Well, she was having midnight picnics before, wasn't she? It was just a different caterer."

In nursing, Ella and I had located each other. Seconds after the doctor tossed her onto my belly, she rooted around and found what she needed. Knowing nothing but what I'd read in books, I followed her lead. *Here you go, Baby. Here you go. Shhhh.* Since then, we had known no other way of being.

But motherhood is about letting go—first from our bodies, then our arms, then our sight, then our homes—and then? Weaning falls hard on this spectrum, forcing me to see the life Ella will live far beyond me, where she will learn to find her own sustenance, her own comfort.

I have never seen a child of mine grow up. I am starting to see what it looks like.

☀

Jill Christman's memoir, *Darkroom: A Family Exposure*, was published in 2002. She teaches writing in Muncie, Indiana, where she lives with her husband, writer Mark Neely, daughter Ella, and son Huck. "Weaning Ella" was originally published in the Spring 2007 issue of *Brain, Child: The Magazine for Thinking Mothers*.

CONTRIBUTORS

Melissa Balmain's writing has appeared in *The New Yorker*, *The New York Times*, *Details*, and other magazines and newspapers, and in anthologies that include *How to Fit a Car Seat on a Camel*. A contributing editor and humorist for *Parenting* and *Babytalk*, she's at work on several books. Her latest postbreastfeeding addiction is Trader Joe's turkey jerky.

Patricia Berry has worked as a writer, columnist, and editor for the past twenty-five years. Her features and columns have appeared in *The New York Times*, *Working Mother*, *New Jersey Life*, *This Old House Magazine*, *ADDitude*, and other publications. Her essay "Unwanted Hair Growth" was published in the 2007 anthology *Over the Hill and Between the Sheets: Sex, Love, and Lust in Middle Age*. A founding editor of *Sports Illustrated for Kids*, Berry is at work on her first novel. She lives in New Jersey with her husband and three daughters.

Jill Christman's memoir, *Darkroom: A Family Exposure*, was published by the University of Georgia Press in 2002 and won the Association of Writers and Writing Programs Award Series in Creative Nonfiction. Her work has been nominated twice for a Pushcart Prize, and her recent essays have appeared in *River Teeth*, *Brevity*, *Mississippi Review*, *Harpur Palate*, *Literary Mama*, and many other journals. She teaches creative nonfiction writing in the MFA program at Ashland University, and she is an associate professor at Ball State University in Muncie, Indiana, where she lives with her husband, writer Mark Neely; daughter Ella; and son Huck. "Weaning Ella" was originally published in the Spring 2007 issue of *Brain, Child: The Magazine for Thinking Mothers*.

Jill Hamburg Coplan began her career as a wire-service and newspaper reporter in the Middle East and Africa. She wrote the "Work & Family" column for BusinessWeek.com. Now she divides her time between editing at *BusinessWeek*, teaching journalism at New York University, freelance magazine writing, and working on a novel—all thanks to her husband, David, and babysitter, Naseem. In her copious spare time she runs after her five- and eight-year-old sons. Her personal website is jillhamburgcoplan.com.

Leslie Crawford is a writer living in San Francisco with her husband, Steve, and two children, Sam and Molly. Crawford is a regular contributor to *San Francisco Magazine* and BabyCenter.com, and she has written for *Metropolis*, *Salon*, *Garden Design*, and other publications.

Alice Elliott Dark is the author of the novel *Think of England* and two collections of short stories, *In the Gloaming* and *Naked to the Waist*. Her short stories have appeared in *The New Yorker*,

Harper's, *Redbook*, *DoubleTake*, *Best American Short Stories*, and *Prize Stories: The O. Henry Awards 2000*, among other publications, and have been translated into many languages. Her story "In the Gloaming" was made into films by HBO and Trinity Playhouse. Her reviews and essays have appeared in *The New York Times*, *The Washington Post*, and many anthologies. She is the writer in residence of the English Department at Rutgers-Newark.

Daryn Eller is a freelance writer whose work has appeared in *Parents*, *Parenting*, *O: The Oprah Magazine*, *Prevention*, and *Health* magazines. She is the coauthor of *Rooms to Grow In: Little Folk Art's Great Rooms for Babies, Kids, and Teens* (Clarkson Potter, 2001). She lives in Venice, California.

Deborah Garrison is the author of the poetry collections *The Second Child* and *A Working Girl Can't Win*. Born in Ann Arbor, Michigan, she worked on the editorial staff of *The New Yorker* for many years and is now an editor at Alfred A. Knopf and Pantheon Books. She lives with her husband and children in Montclair, New Jersey.

Ann Matturro Gault spent a decade on the staff of *Family Circle* magazine before deciding to freelance full time in 2000 (when baby number three was born). She has written about parenting, health, and education for many publications, including *Redbook, Reader's Digest, First for Women*, and Scholastic.com. Gault's blog about life as a mother of elementary-school kids currently appears each week on Scholastic.com. She lives with her husband and their four children in a boring New Jersey suburb but vows to return to Manhattan as soon as she gets the chance.

Julia Glass is the author of the novels *The Whole World Over* and *Three Junes*, which won the 2002 National Book Award for Fiction. Her third work of fiction, *I See You Everywhere*, was published by Pantheon Books in 2008. She has received fellowships from the National Endowment for the Arts, the New York Foundation for the Arts, and the Radcliffe Institute for Advanced Study. She has also won the Tobias Wolff Award, three Nelson Algren fiction awards, the Roy T. Ames Memorial Essay Award, and the Pirate's Alley Faulkner Society medal for Best Novella. She lives in Massachusetts with her family.

Stephanie Kilroy graduated from the University of California, Los Angeles, with a degree in history. She also studied creative writing, and one of her plays, *Junk Hungry*, was produced in Los Angeles. She writes in Reno, Nevada, where she lives with her husband, Brian, and her four children, Leilani, Zoey-Cate, Leo, and Dominic.

Pamela Kruger is a freelance writer, editor, and blogger whose work has been published in *The New York Times*, *Child*, *Parenting*, *Fast Company*, *The Huffington Post*, and other publications. Her essays have appeared in several anthologies, including *A Love Like No Other: Stories from Adoptive Parents*, which she coedited with Jill Smolowe. Kruger lives with her husband and their two daughters in New Jersey.

Fernanda Moore has written for numerous publications, including *New York Magazine*, *The New York Times Magazine*, and *Parenting*, and she is a regular book reviewer for the *Nashville Scene*. She has finally finished her dissertation on an obscure

Byzantine poem (part of the dissertation appears in the anthology *Classics and National Cultures*) and has completed her Ph.D. in comparative literature from Stanford University. She lives with her family in Swarthmore, Pennsylvania.

Catherine Newman, author of the award-winning memoir *Waiting for Birdy*, is a contributing editor at *FamilyFun* and *Wondertime* magazines and a regular contributor to *O, The Oprah Magazine*. She writes a weekly parenting column, "The Dalai Mama," at Wondertime.com, and she wrote the column "Bringing Up Ben and Birdy" for BabyCenter.com. Her work has been published in numerous magazines and anthologies, including *The Bitch in the House*, a *New York Times* bestseller. She lives in Massachusetts with her (entirely weaned) family.

Dawn Porter, who served for five years as director of news practices for ABC News, is now vice president of standards and practices at the A&E Television Networks. Porter is currently at work on a biography of nineteenth-century African American suffragist and civil-rights pioneer Ida Wells-Barnett. She and her husband, David Graff, live in Montclair, New Jersey, with their two adorable sons.

Heidi Raykeil is the author of *Confessions of a Naughty Mommy: How I Found My Lost Libido* (thenaughtymommy.com). Her writing has been featured in *Parenting* magazine and online at *Literary Mama*. She is a contributor to several anthologies and collaborative projects, including *Literary Mama: Reading for the Maternally Inclined; Using Our Words: Moms and Dads on Raising Kids in the Neighborhood*, and the new *Our Bodies, Ourselves: Pregnancy and Birth*. She lives in Seattle with her family.

Jessica Restaino is an assistant professor of English at Montclair State University. Her scholarly work focuses on preparation of new teachers, writing pedagogy, and the political thought of Hannah Arendt. She is the proud mother of Abby.

Maura Rhodes is a contributing editor for *Parenting* magazine, where she was a senior editor for nine and a half years. She is the author of several books, including *Radu's Simply Fit*, with celebrity trainer Radu Teodorescu, and *Baby Must-Haves: The Essential Guide to Everything from Cribs to Bibs*. Her personal essays appear in *It's a Boy: Women Writers on Raising Sons* and *My Father Married Your Mother: Writers Talk about Stepparents, Stepchildren, and Everyone in Between*. Other writing credits include articles for such publications as *Redbook*, *Good Housekeeping*, *McCall's*, *Women's Sports and Fitness*, *Real Simple*, *Self*, and *Parenting*. Rhodes lives in Montclair, New Jersey, with her husband and four children. Her breast pump currently resides in her garage-sale pile.

Rachel Sarah, a year into single motherhood, stopped picking up toys and started picking up men. Not really—her life is actually quite tame. Her book *Single Mom Seeking: Playdates, Blind Dates and Other Dispatches from the Dating World* was published in 2007 by Seal Press/Avalon. She has also written for *Family Circle*, *Pregnancy*, *Parenting*, *Literary Mama*, BabyCenter.com, and *American Baby*. Rachel is the single-mom columnist for LifetimeTV.com. Please visit her at singlemomseeking.com.

Suzanne Schlosberg earns her living as both a humorist and a health writer. She is the author of *The Curse of the Singles Table: A True Story of 1001 Nights without Sex*, and her essays have appeared in anthologies such as *Sand in My Bra and Other Misadventures; Whose Panties Are These?*; and *Single State of the Union*. On the health front, she is the author of *The Essential Fertility Log* and *The Ultimate Workout Log* and coauthor of *The Essential Breastfeeding Log, Fitness for Dummies, and Weight Training for Dummies*. Suzanne lives with her husband and twin sons in Bend, Oregon, and can be reached at suzanneschlosberg.com.

Paula Spencer is the author of *Momfidence! An Oreo Never Killed Anybody and Other Secrets of Happier Parenting*, the "Momfidence" columnist for *Woman's Day* magazine, and a longtime contributing editor of *Parenting* and *Babytalk*. She has collaborated on eight books concerning pregnancy, parenting, and health, including *Bright from the Start* and *The Happiest Toddler on the Block*. As a founding contributing editor of Caring.com, she has extended her expertise from growing kids to aging parents. She lives with her husband and their four children in Chapel Hill, North Carolina.

Dana Sullivan has written for *The New York Times, O: The Oprah Magazine, Real Simple, More, Outside, Self, Health, Parenting*, and *Parents*, among other publications. She is a contributing writer for *Shape's Fit Pregnancy*. *Unbuttoned* is her second collaboration with Maureen Connolly; they co-wrote *The Essential C-Section Guide*, which was published by Broadway Books/Random House in 2004. Dana has a degree in English literature from the University of California, Los Angeles. She lives in Reno, Nevada, with her husband, Robert Kilroy, and their three children, Liam, Julia, and Carina. Dana is working on her first novel and can be reached by email at Danasullivan@mac.com.

Rebecca Walker is an award-winning, best-selling author and speaker who has contributed to the global conversation about identity, power, and the need for human evolution for over fifteen years. Her books include *To Be Real: Telling the Truth and Changing the Face of Feminism; Black, White, and Jewish: Autobiography of a Shifting Self*; and *Baby Love: Choosing Motherhood After a Lifetime of Ambivalence*. Her essays, articles, and reviews appear regularly in blogs, magazines, and popular anthologies. She lectures widely and teaches the art of the memoir in MFA programs and workshops around the world. Contact Walker via her personal website: rebeccawalker.com.

Nancy M. Williams, after weaning her daughter, went on to lead Virgin Mobile USA's e-commerce sales and marketing group. She and her team (which included a nursing mother) increased VMU's online sales in pace with the company's own spectacular growth rate. In late 2006 Williams took a sabbatical from her twenty-year marketing career to focus on creative writing. Since then, her work has appeared in *Fit Pregnancy* and *New Jersey Family* magazines. Ms. Williams lives in Montclair, New Jersey, with her husband, David, and her two children. Gracie, now six, still remembers nursing.

Rachel Zucker is the author of three books of poetry: *The Bad Wife Handbook, The Last Clear Narrative*, and *Eating in the Underworld*. Along with the poet Arielle Greenberg, she is coeditor of an anthology of essays, *Women Poets on Mentorship: Efforts and Affections*, published by the University of Iowa Press in 2008, and coauthor of a book-length lyric essay, *Home/Birth*. Zucker has taught poetry and writing at several universities, including New York University and Yale, and was the poet in residence at Fordham for two years. She is also a certified labor doula. Zucker lives in New York City with her husband, Josh Goren, and their three sons. For more information visit her website: rachelzucker.net.

*For a list of discussion group questions and a link to the
Facebook online community for continuing the conversation,
please visit www.unbuttonedbook.com.*

If you or someone you know are looking for helpful references on the subject of breast-feeding, or if you are nursing and need some guidance, these books from The Harvard Common Press are a valuable resource.

Harvard Common Press books are available wherever books are sold. To learn more about Harvard Common Press parenting and childcare titles, please visit our website, www.harvardcommonpress.com.

The Nursing Mother's Companion
20th Anniversary Edition
by Kathleen Huggins, R.N., M.S.
$14.95 paperback, ISBN 978-1-55832-304-9
The fifth edition of this best-selling, widely acclaimed guide for nursing mothers has been completely revised and updated. In addition to covering all the basics of breast-feeding, the book includes an extensive index on the safety of drugs during breastfeed-ing and "survival guide" sections to help nursing mothers quickly identify and solve problems during each stage of breastfeeding.

The Nursing Mother's Guide to Weaning
*How to Bring the Breastfeeding to a Gentle Close,
and How to Decide When the Time Is Right*
by Kathleen Huggins, R.N., M.S., and Linda Ziedrich
$11.95 paperback, ISBN 978-1-55832-352-0
This revised edition provides invaluable advice on a subject that has caused distress for countless mothers—when and how to wean—with guidance on the safest, least stress-ful ways to bring breastfeeding to a gentle close at every age, from early infancy through toddlerhood and beyond.

Nursing Mother, Working Mother
The Essential Guide to Breastfeeding Your Baby Before and After You Return to Work
by Gale Pryor
$12.95 paperback, ISBN 978-1-55832-331-5
With straightforward information and an encouraging tone, Pryor advises working mothers who want to continue breastfeeding on everything from how to simplify life at home to how to maintain one's milk supply, pump breast milk at work, and store and transport breast milk safely and conveniently.

25 Things Every Nursing Mother Needs to Know
by Kathleen Huggins, R.N., M.S., and Jan Ellen Brown
$12.95 hardcover, ISBN 978-1-55832-383-4
This concise, inspirational guide provides all the essential information on breastfeeding for mothers-to-be and new moms in an attractive, easy-to-use package. In a friendly, support-ive tone, the authors discuss such topics as latching on, soothing a fussy baby, choosing a breast pump, balancing work and breastfeeding, introducing solid foods, and much more.